WOMEN ACTION TAKERS WHO GAINED BY LOSING

Inspirational and Motivational Stories from Women Who Use Intermittent Fasting and Will NEVER DIET AGAIN!

Curated by

Paige Davidson, Laurie Lewis, and Star McEuen

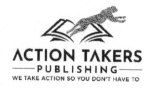

ACTION TAKERS
—PUBLISHING—
WE TAKE ACTION SO YOU DON'T HAVE TO

Action Takers Publishing™
San Diego, California

Action Takers Publishing™
www.actiontakerspublishing.com

ebook ISBN: 978-1-956665-06-2
Paperback ISBN: 978-1-956665-05-5

100% of the net proceeds of the sales of this book will be donated to a 501(c)(3) nonprofit charity.

Cover Design by Sam Art Studio
Printed in the United States of America

TABLE OF CONTENTS

"See yourself through the eyes of others, for others see the real you."

~Lynda Sunshine West

FOREWORD

Dr. Bert Herring
Author of AC: The Power of Appetite Correction

This book encourages you by sharing others' real-life experiences as you begin your new fat-loss/weight-maintenance lifestyle. Look at the word "encourage." It's "en" plus "courage," meaning "put courage in."

Why does starting a new weight loss effort require courage? Is it dangerous? Is it frightening?

The health benefits of losing surplus fat are the opposite of dangerous. However, starting a new fat-loss effort can be truly frightening, because for most, it isn't the first try. Maybe you've tried one or two or forty different ways. Maybe you've tried eat-less-exercise-more without seeing a sustainable loss. Maybe you've read lots of success stories but doubt your dream of similar success can come true. Maybe you've spent thousands of dollars on various plans and programs. Maybe, like Paige, you've tried surgery. Fear of failure with a new fat-loss plan may not be Stephen King frightening, but overcoming the fear takes courage.

That's why Paige, Laurie, and Star are encouraging you with these "results typical" success stories. These accounts describe big successes and little ones. They're real-life accounts from people like you with similar challenges: families, work, budgets and other obligations. They're not Hollywood actors, elite athletes, reality show participants or full-time bodybuilders. They're people sharing their stories because not long ago, they stood where you stand now: highly motivated to lose fat and afraid—yes, afraid—of putting themselves on another path to failure—another waste of time, money, and effort. They want you to know what worked for them and how they dealt with obstacles. They want you to learn from their successes—and mistakes! These stories will help you move ahead with appropriate expectations so you can write your own fat-loss success story. Their common theme? Success with Intermittent Fasting/time restricted eating (IF/TRE) is common!

Common, but not guaranteed. IF/TRE isn't perfect. Since writing my first book on the subject in 2005, I've been looking for ways to spot the few people for whom it's not going to work. There's still no magic answer, but IF/TRE remains the most powerful and reliable weight loss tool I've ever seen. Each of the real-life stories Paige, Laurie, and Star have collected in this book offers a reason to have courage—the courage you need to pick up this tool and put your energy and confidence behind it.

Everyone is different, so your success story—and the rewards you appreciate most—will be unique. This book's title speaks to all that can be gained by losing. As you make your way through this book, I invite you to anticipate which reward you will value most. Will it be a gain, such as freedom, power and control over food and appetite? Or a loss—a vanishing health problem, fading work and social bias, or losing a negative self-image? What will your story be?

A SUNNY NOTE FROM PAIGE DAVIDSON, LAURIE LEWIS, AND STAR MCEUEN

The dieting industry in the United States is big business. In 2020 alone, the U.S. weight-loss industry was valued at $71 billion (Healthline Media). Sadly, the dieters paying all this money have a collective 95% failure rate. Yes, you read that figure correctly. Diet culture, diet mentality, and social media influences all result in women feeling they need to be thin to be attractive, to fit in, to be socially acceptable, to be taken seriously.

Yet there is a solution to weight loss and reclaiming health that is absolute freedom from dieting! Certified Intermittent Fasting Health Coaches Paige Davidson and Laurie Lewis, and Intermittent Fasting Accountability Coach Star McEuen have all discovered the health practice of Intermittent Fasting and never looked back. The practice changed our lives in a lasting and profound way.

After learning about Intermittent Fasting, Laurie lost over 50 pounds after several years in menopause hell. Paige, after 40+ years of yo-yo dieting and even unsuccessful weight loss surgery, discovered Intermittent Fasting and lost 110 pounds and cured several obesity-related health conditions. Star, who also tried diet after diet for many years, unsuccessfully, discovered Intermittent Fasting and lost an incredible 81 pounds.

All of us became acquainted through the virtual international Intermittent Fasting community and soon grew to respect each other greatly. We have a goal of helping as many women as possible in discovering the amazing health benefits of the practice of Intermittent Fasting.

All three of us have been featured on multiple podcasts and social media events for our personal success and knowledge of Intermittent Fasting. Eventually we realized that a book featuring real success stories of intermittent fasters would be an amazing way to encourage and motivate women globally in reclaiming their own personal health and vitality, as well as in losing weight if that was their goal.

This collection of Intermittent Fasting success stories was lovingly curated by the three of us. Each story is unique. Success means something different to each of the women who share their deeply personal journeys. You will read inspiring stories from women of all ages, from the mid-30s through 85 years young! Some of these women have battled obesity their entire lives. Some were a very healthy weight, then battled the ravages of menopause successfully through their Intermittent Fasting practices. Some have lost large amounts of weight while others lost a modest amount of weight and gained wellness in other forms. None of the authors are physicians or nutritionists. Each result is unique to each author.

We, along with the women represented within this book, are proud to share the lessons learned, the hard-won experiences in taking back our lives, and the joy and contentment that comes with living a healthy lifestyle with the side effect of weight loss!

NOTE: The information in this book is not intended or implied to be a substitute for professional medical advice, diagnosis, or treatment. Always consult your physician before beginning any exercise or diet program. These stories are not intended to diagnose any medical condition or to replace your healthcare professional. Consult with your healthcare professional to design an appropriate diet and exercise prescription.

With Gratitude,
Paige Davidson, Laurie Lewis, and Star McEuen

Chapter 1

A WEIGHT LOSS JOURNEY IS A SPIRITUAL JOURNEY WITH HOLISTIC HEALING

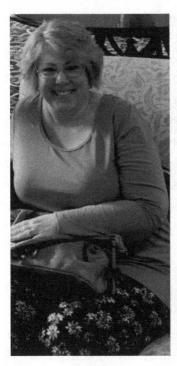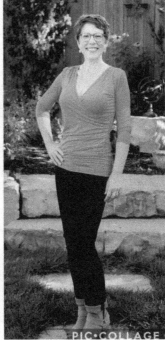

by Paige Davidson

My 8-hour shift at the public library was nearing an end when a beloved regular patron, an intelligent, spry, 85-year-old woman, asked for help faxing a document. It was a very simple task, but my desire to assist her was twinged with anxiety. *The fax workstation is at the opposite end of the building,* I thought. *I don't know if I'll be able to make it all the way there and back.* My knees and feet had been hurting terribly for the past two hours. As the customer and I set off for the fax workstation, sure enough, the pain became too much to endure, and I fell behind. At 249 pounds, my weight was exacerbating the arthritis and inflammation in my knees, along with the plantar fasciitis in my right foot and the Achilles tendonitis in my left foot. With each step, I struggled unsuccessfully not to grimace in pain, and tears began to pool in my eyes. *I truly love this job, but I can barely do it anymore,* I thought. *I can't keep on going this way; something has to change!* At that moment, all I could do was pray that God would help me make it, and thankfully He did.

On the drive home from work that night, the tears flowed in earnest. So many feelings roiled within me: embarrassment, panic, pain, exhaustion, frustration, and, sadly, familiarity with having been here before. A shocking realization swept over me – if something didn't change, I was in danger of needing a walker to be able to work, or even just to get around. At 56 years old, this notion hit me like a punch to the gut. At this point, I didn't even know where to begin to make changes, but little did I know that the answer was there within the library walls. My last prayer before I arrived at home was for God to somehow help me be able to walk without pain.

How he was going to do that was surely a mystery to me. Clearly, I had to lose weight – yet again. But at this point in my life, I had given up on diets. The knowledge that my health depended on my losing weight felt like the weight of the world on my shoulders.

A Sad History

I grew up in a diet culture, both in my home and in society. I learned early on that in order to lose weight, you had to "go somewhere." Some diet doctor had to fix you, to tell you what to do, what to eat and not eat. For most of my life, beginning as a young teen, I tried every weight loss center in existence, falling into a vicious cycle that would continue until my mid-fifties. Join, full of hope that this was going to be the time that I would finally lose the weight and look skinny and gorgeous. I would try my very best and lose weight! But over time, the restrictions began to make it harder and harder to comply with the many rules of the diet; weighing my food, keeping journals, counting calories or micros & macros, the elimination of entire food groups, eating foods only from the "good foods" list, and trying to stay away from the "bad foods" list. Until finally, I would quit the diet in frustration and embarrassment. Next, I would return to eating how I was before, and the weight would return plus more. I would say I was finished dieting, until the next time someone called me fat, or ignored me in a situation that particularly stung, or I got so winded trying to climb a single flight of stairs that it scared me, and there I would go again, off to join yet another weight loss program. The cycle would begin again, the same process playing itself out as my self-esteem continued to plummet, until it was practically non-existent.

Years later, after dieting my way up to 315 pounds, I finally tried the ultimate weight loss strategy, dreaded weight loss surgery. At age 37, I was the second Roux-en-Y gastric bypass patient in Kentucky in 2000. The procedure was so new, the hospital wasn't fully prepared. When the nurse came to get me from the recovery room with a regular sized wheelchair to take me to my hospital room, I took one look at it and knew immediately that there was no way I could fit into it. I tried and, sure enough, I was far too big to be able to sit in it. I had to walk from the recovery room to my hospital room. The nurse was amazed that I was able to do it, but talk about humiliation! Right before he operated on me, the surgeon said "Paige, I can operate on your stomach, but I can't operate on your brain." And that was it. There was no further assistance or information in this area. I was given this amazing new tool to help me lose weight, but was not given what I needed most.

Clearly there was something wrong with my thinking, but what? When you have thought the same way since you were a child, you believe that is just the way it is. How everyone thinks. What is normal. I absolutely could not identify how my thinking was flawed, or caused me to gain, then lose, then gain, ad nauseam. The first step in healing is always awareness. How can you heal from disordered thinking, if you have no idea that your thinking is disordered? Providing me with the physical tool to assist me in losing weight yet failing to provide me with the tools to change my lifestyle, mindset, attitude, and disordered thinking was tantamount to failing me. And yet, who did I blame when after losing 150 pounds, and keeping it off for about five years, I gained most of that weight back? Myself, of course! Never mind that if I had known how to 'cure' myself all on my own, I would never have been morbidly obese in the first place. My growing sense of failure continued to snowball, and this is how I wound up back up to 249 pounds at age 56, dangerously close to being disabled by arthritis and inflammation.

Answered Prayers

If you recall, I had prayed for God to help me just be able to walk without pain. He answered that prayer in two ways. First, he led me to do something that I had never done, in all those attempts to lose weight. He led me to seek Christian counseling. I was finished chasing skinny, and I was ready to figure out what my issues were that kept me morbidly obese all those years. Now, I wanted something new, because so much more than my looks mattered now. What was at stake was my health, my sanity, and my future. What I was seeking was holistic wellness; physical, emotional, mental, and spiritual. I wanted to be in healthy alignment in all areas of my life. I prayed about finding a great Christian counselor and was able to do just that.

While Linda and I got to work getting to know each other, and praying for God's grace and assistance, God answered my prayer in a second way. My sister shared with me that she was doing something called Intermittent Fasting. I had never heard of it before and asked her for details. When she shared that she ate her food within a certain number of hours per day, and the rest of the time she fasted – she ate nothing at all, I stopped her. "That sounds like some kind of fad diet, and I am never dieting again!" I told her. She laughed and said it isn't a diet, and it isn't a fad. Fasting has been around for thousands of years. I still dismissed her, until she said that the reason she had shared was because she knew how much pain I was in. Intermittent fasting heals inflammation, and she thought it might help my pain. Now that got my attention! The very next day at work a patron returned a book called *Delay, Don't Deny: Living an Intermittent Fasting Lifestyle* by Gin Stephens. To this day, I know that the Lord placed this book in my hands. It was the beginning of the life change and holistic wellness that I had prayed for.

To practice Intermittent Fasting is simply to eat within a time period each day. Typically, one would start out slowly, by fasting either 14 hours and eating 10 hours, called 14/10, or fasting 16 hours and eating 8 hours, aka 16/8. The consecutive hours that you eat each day is called your eating window. Intermittent fasting is not a diet and does not address what you eat – that is completely up to you – but addresses when you eat.

Because I was desperate to heal my pain, I didn't ease into fasting, I jumped right in at a healing protocol of 19 hours of fasting for one week and then moved to a 20-hour fast. At the end of two weeks, the next miracle came. Although I still had foot pain, my pain was reduced so significantly that I was able to walk normally. No limping, after just two weeks! I was so grateful to God for this, that I realized I had to keep on going. I practiced 20/4 for three months and had learned from further research that extended protocols are appropriate if you need extra healing. Since I was still experiencing pain, I decided to add in an extended fast every week. I continued with my 20/4 protocol and added in one 43-hour fast each week. It was hard at first, but I got used to it. After an additional 3 months of this protocol, the NEXT miracle occurred: I was completely pain free! Not only had I healed the inflammation in my knee, but the plantar fasciitis and the Achilles tendonitis were 100% healed. And, unbelievably, I had lost almost 60 pounds in that six months of practicing Intermittent Fasting.

Holistic Wellness at Last

Ultimately, I lost 110 pounds in 14 months by living an Intermittent Fasting lifestyle. I have now been an intermittent faster for over three years and will do so for the rest of my life. Not only did I heal the conditions mentioned above, but I also healed my obstructive sleep apnea. I banished the brain fog that had plagued me and increased my energy exponentially. My skin became practically flawless, and no-one can believe that I am 59 years old. To practice Intermittent Fasting is literally to age in reverse! There are so many health benefits to living this lifestyle it is hard to comprehend. And those are just the physical health benefits.

The biggest part of the work that I did was to heal my emotional health. I learned over time to make mindset shifts that would set me up for success rather than failure. I learned what it truly meant to love myself. After engaging in horrible, negative and punitive self-talk since my teen years, I learned how to turn that around. I learned to be kind and loving to myself, to show myself grace when I wasn't perfect in my food choices, and most of all I learned to tell myself the truth. I was not a failure! I absolutely could make good healthy food and beverage choices for myself. Telling myself the truth really did set me free from the emotional bondage that I had been ensnared in for so many years. An important lesson I learned is that we believe what we tell ourselves, no matter if it is positive or negative. So, we must be honest and truthful with ourselves, rather than telling ourselves things out of negative emotions that aren't true. More mindset shifts that helped create true emotional health for me were to learn the importance of being positive, and that being positive is a choice that we make every day. Practicing Intermittent Fasting gave me the space to do this extremely important mindset work, whereas before I was always consumed with food; when was the next meal, what sounded good, when was my next snack, what would it be, etc. I spent so much time obsessing about food that I had no time or space left over to do any work on myself. I also discovered through this lifestyle that I truly had been a food addict, and I learned that there are physicians who prescribe Intermittent Fasting to cure food addiction. I am living proof that it works!

These mindset shifts also served to strengthen my mental health. I found that as I lost weight and felt better physically and emotionally, the depression that I had dealt with for years began to slowly lift. My doctor took me off one medication for depression completely and considerably reduced the dose of a second medication for depression. My mental health is at a good place, and a big part of it is practicing gratitude. I have learned to have a daily gratitude practice, and it is a calming and spiritual part of my day.

Most importantly, my spiritual health has been strengthened, and I have grown so much closer in my relationship with Jesus. As I was losing the weight, I was also learning to pray more, to just talk to God and pour out my heart to him. I also learned to listen to what he was saying to me, in that small feeling that I should do something or do something differently. It really took some practice to listen to those thoughts that entered my mind and know that thought was not on accident. Spiritual growth is so personal and hard for me to explain, but I just developed a closer relationship with Jesus and came to appreciate how good He has been to me. This was a nice cycle to be in. The more I prayed and paid attention, the more I understood what God was saying to me. And the more I understood what He was saying to me, the closer I felt my relationship with Him was growing. As a Christian, this is the most heartwarming effect of my journey. What I thought was a weight-loss journey, turned out to be a spiritual journey with physical, emotional, and mental healing.

Blessed to Pass it On

When I finally achieved holistic wellness, there was just no end to my appreciation and gratitude. I prayed that God would somehow use me to help other women. Women who had yo-yo dieted their whole lives. Women who had experienced the shame and disappointment of a failed weight-loss surgery. Women who reached menopause and felt that this was it. That they were going to have a spare tire and brain fog forever. God helped me in all these circumstances, by bringing the miracle of Intermittent Fasting into my life. So, my prayer was to be able to pass it on, to help as many women as possible through my experiences.

And did He ever! He led me to become a certified health/life coach. I started a virtual coaching business, focusing on Intermittent Fasting and mindset shifts. Life became a whirlwind of blessings! I didn't know how to reach out and help other women, so God led the way. He opened doors for me and presented me with options and possibilities that I never even knew existed. He led me to accept the following opportunities, all in the interest of helping as many women as possible achieve the amazing health that I had been blessed with through Intermittent Fasting:

✓ I moved from being a member of 12 different private Facebook® Intermittent Fasting support groups to being a moderator in those groups…inspiring, mentoring, coaching, and educating others, with a combined group membership of over half a million people.

✓ I moderate my own inspirational Facebook® page called The Fasting PAIGE, with over one thousand follows.

✓ I started offering a free virtual weekly class to seniors, called Intermittent Fasting 101, through an app called Lindy.

✓ I joined a social media platform called Clubhouse and offer free Intermittent Fasting education and coaching to a worldwide audience.

✓ I have now been a guest on 14 different podcasts and Facebook® Live events, sharing my knowledge and experience with Intermittent Fasting.

✓ I have become an author, contributing various iterations of my Intermittent Fasting story to five different anthology books, one workbook on Intermittent Fasting, and am in the process of writing my story mixed with information to educate others about Intermittent Fasting.

✓ I have been invited to be a panelist for five different virtual summits to share my Intermittent Fasting story and experience as a coach, an author, and an expert on healing inflammation through Intermittent Fasting.

✓ I was featured on the cover of *Woman's World* magazine in 2020 (an international magazine with a readership of 1.6 million in the U.S. alone), and in 2021 I was featured in a special edition of *Women's World* magazine, *Half Their Size Over 50!*

✓ I am a member of an ongoing anti-bullying panel to shed light on the effects of bullying, remedies, and prevention through Relentless & Unstoppable, a virtual group with an international audience.

✓ I am a co-host on the Thriving Women Network show Uncomfortable Conversations, and occasional co-host on the shows Book-ish Talk and Thriving Women Talk. These programs are offered virtually via e360tv, a streaming network offering content in culture, healthy living, independent entertainment, extreme sports, fresh perspectives, and cannabis.

While I don't really know what it looks like, I'm so excited about what the future holds, and my weight is no longer going to stop me from achieving success.

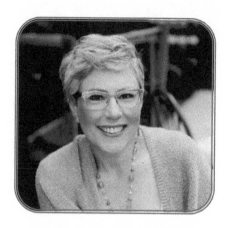

PAIGE DAVIDSON

Paige Davidson is a certified health and life coach specializing in Intermittent Fasting and mindset shifts. She holds a BA and MA in education and worked for the state of Kentucky as a trainer, workshop facilitator, communications specialist, and executive staff advisor for a state agency head. After taking early retirement and having to have a knee replacement at only 56-years old, she took her health into her own hands and lost 110 pounds with Intermittent Fasting. As the Founder of Fasting with Paige, her professional goal is to help as many women as possible lose weight and achieve holistic wellness.

As a certified health coach, I would be honored and excited to help you learn the ins-and-outs of Intermittent Fasting, and to guide and support you as you work toward holistic health for yourself!

Connect with Paige at https://fastingwithpaige.com/.

Chapter 2

MAGICAL QUESTIONS

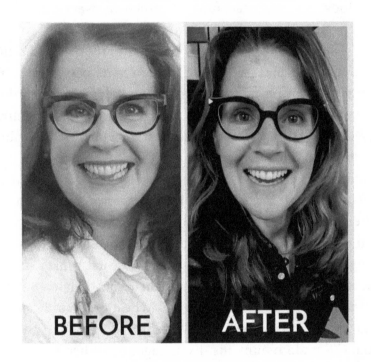

BEFORE   AFTER

by Laurie Lewis

Standing at the sink in her sunny kitchen, I completely lost it, ranting and wailing like a furious 5-year-old.

What she'd asked was, "Shall we use this time that you're home to turn the weight around?"

I wasn't 5. I was 54 and had just about given up all hope. I was in pain from head to toe, my equilibrium was off, memory loss and brain fog were debilitating, and I'd put on 50 pounds of stubborn, menopausal weight.

"MOM! You don't understand. I've tried everything. I can't just snap my fingers and turn it around. What am I supposed to do? I'm the healthiest eater anyone knows, I take good care of myself, and it makes no difference. I want to feel like myself again. I can't just 'turn it around'; I've been trying for almost five years."

She looked at me peacefully. Breathed in everything I'd said, and responded, "Laurie Love. Let's pray for an answer." Willingly accepting her kindness, I trudged upstairs to tuck in. I had nearly resigned to getting heavier, foggier, and in more pain forever. Fearful thoughts crept in, "Maybe it really is all downhill from here?" Yet, even though I felt despondent, I had enough remaining hope to curl up in bed and search for "menopausal stubborn fat weight loss help!" one final time.

"Final time," because the answer came. I'd heard about long, therapeutic fasting, but never knew that a person could adopt "Intermittent Fasting" as a daily health practice. This unfamiliar term popped up in my search, which astounded me because I had been studying nutrition and health for over 20 years. What's this? You choose a time to fast every day, and then consolidate your meals into an eating window? I figured it had to be more complicated than that. So, I read, listened, studied all night, and as the sun peeked up over the Colorado mountains, I was eager to let her know I might have discovered an answer.

I shared bits of what I'd absorbed overnight – you eat in an eating window, don't take in any nutrients while fasting, and it balances your hormones and taps into excess body fat for fuel. I said I wanted to try it and assured her, "If I feel sick, I'll quit right away. Or, if I act impatient, grumpy, or mean, you can tell me to stop." She responded with the most assuring words, "How may I support you?"

"Um, I guess… don't offer me breakfast?" That was Day One, and here I am, five years later having chosen to fast clean and eat in an eating window every day. The results feel impressive. I lost 51 pounds in 15 months, fit back into the clothes I love, my skin is smooth, hair and nails grow quickly, plantar fasciitis disappeared, my eyesight improved, dental cleanings are quick, gum health is better, and a large cyst on my spine went away. I have no aches and pains, recover quickly from workouts, and sleep soundly. At 59 years old, my hormones are in balance, and I feel better than I did at 29.

Yet, in the beginning, I couldn't have known that any of that would happen. What I did know, is that standing in that very same kitchen three days later, I had a very strange feeling. I was clear. Things seemed bright. I was settled into my body and had a soothing sense of confidence. The thought came, I feel like myself again. Myself.

It's hard to put words to what feeling like yourself feels like. It's a familiar remembering, but it's new. It's fresh, and light, and quiet. That's when I knew Intermittent Fasting was something sacred. It's not a diet; it's a quiet.

Sure, there were days over the year that followed when I was bored, resentful, impatient, and feeling sorry for myself. But those moments were fleeting compared to feeling energetic, focused, happy, determined, and liberated.

In the early months, I looked to the clock as my target. I had the aim of first 16 hours, then 18, then 20, but I very soon used "Feeling Good" as my guide. Sometimes I barely made it to 12 hours, and other times I fasted 40 hours.

Because my daily fasting felt supremely natural, as my body was designed, I learned what real hunger does and doesn't feel like, discovered which foods make me feel amazing and which do not. I tuned into how my body is healing at certain fasting intervals and how I was feeling refreshed and fully alive during the clean fasting hours.

Five Questions / Five Years

After keeping an eating window every day for five years, I can see that my sacred ritual is grounded in five questions. I consistently ask myself...

1. When am I eating today?

Every day, without fail, I choose to eat in an eating window. This begins with having a sense of when it will be. I look ahead in my calendar, plan out groceries and meals, think about a delicious snack I'll eat to open my window, and enjoy the day in a fasted state. Some days, hunger waves come on a little stronger, but because I know the difference between "real" hunger and a short wave, I ride it out and fast forward!

I first learned to ask this question when I was traveling and thought I could take some days off from fasting. I had been practicing I.F. for two months and my travel schedule seemed complicated. However, I was worried that if I stopped, I might never start again. So, I sat with my calendar and decided when my eating window would be each day. Even though the time shifted, my focus and determination did not. I knew right then that I could have an eating window every day, no matter what life threw at me.

2. Am I experiencing this "hunger" feeling because I'm sleep deprived, stressed, hurt, annoyed, bored, anxious, sad, avoiding something, or think I deserve a reward?

As Gin Stephens, mama-bear of the clean fast, writes, "Hunger is not an emergency" in her bestselling book, *Delay, Don't Deny*. I pause and ask myself, what kind of "hunger" is this? As soon as I recognize it for what it is, I can thank my body for doing its job so well, and I (usually) choose to fast forward and open my eating window later.

Popping food into my mouth to solve some sort of problem was a mindless habit. It took me nearly a year to easily discern what was happening with my emotions, mind, and body that was having me automatically reach for food when I wasn't actually hungry. Knowing *when* my eating window opens and knowing *what* yumminess I'll be eating helps to quiet the temptation of mindless eating.

It dawned on me that my ancestors didn't have a snack an arm's length away to deal with every upset or boredom, so I can certainly bring some awareness and patience to whatever I'm dealing with. I don't need to eat my troubles away. Breathe.

3. Given what I have going on for the next few hours, will I feel my best in a Fed or Fasted state?

Sometimes I'm faced with an unexpected activity, or I feel overwhelmed, or I have an important presentation, or my belly is making ridiculous noises! I begin with the acknowledgment that I can *always* choose to eat.

Old diet-mindset would have me think that's some sort of failure. Nonsense! I tune into what my body is telling me and look at what my schedule informs me I'm up to. Then I imagine what it would feel like to eat now, and what it would feel like to keep fasting. Which choice will have me feel productive and energetic? Then I choose! Fed or Fasted? Both are fabulous options, and one will serve me better right now.

I learned to ask this question during a scary situation on an airplane a few years ago. The pilot informed us that we would need to do an emergency landing, and as we made our approach the firetrucks and ambulances lined the runway. Thankfully, the plane functioned correctly, but when I got safely into the airport my body SCREAMED for FOOD. EAT NOW.

That was puzzling because it was 6:00 a.m. and I hadn't eaten at that time in years. I made the very real correlation between stress and the body demanding food and I gave myself a choice. "Sure, go eat now! It's fine. But who knows how long I'll be in this airport and when I'll ultimately reach my destination? So, will I feel better Fed or Fasted?" The answer was obvious. My body told me to keep fasting. It always knows.

4. What delicious food does my body need/want today?

Because my body is healing during the fasting hours, it is now extra communicative in terms of the foods it needs and doesn't want. I can look in the fridge or at a menu and my body will steer me towards the nutrients it needs. It will also let me know which foods it's "not interested in." That's what it actually says! "Nope, not interested. Not that, not that, not that... That!" Or, I'll have strong communication from my body that it wants (fill in the blank) for days! It needs those nutrients and it's nudging me.

This discernment is a result of daily clean fasting. It's the ultimate "intuitive eating" because I can hear what my body is telling me. I am not trying to "be good," like a restrictive diet; my body is supremely interested in feeling good. One of my mantras is, "It's not about being good; it's about feeling good."

Dr. Bert Herring describes this memorably when he envisions animals in the wild and their innate ability to know what to eat and when to stop eating. His book, *AC: The Power of Appetite Correction* came to life for me when I was in South Africa and saw two cheetahs chasing down an impala. Who knows how many hours they had been out there trying? They sure earned that feast.

Eating slowly, they sat up after a while, licked each other off as kitties do, and sauntered away from their half-eaten dinner. Their bodies informed them that they were satisfied, finished, and they didn't need to clean their plate. That's Appetite Correction in action!

I also make sure that if I'm heading to an event that I'll open my eating window early and eat exactly what my body needs today. I'm also considering quantity. Who knows what little bits of food they are going to feed me at an event, and some days my body is extremely hungry. So, I always eat ahead of time, even if that means eating a bit earlier than planned.

Listening in this way came gradually. I noticed that if I was scrambling and didn't plan or listen to my body, that it often got puffy, achy, groggy, ravenous, moody, annoyed, and dissatisfied after I ate. But, if I consistently tune into the foods that make my body happy, it serves me well, and I am happy!

5. What can I do to take really good care of myself right now?

I realized that I crash and burn when I take on too much or have complicated, aggressive plans to improve myself. There is too much to think about! Fasting, nutrition, meditation & prayer, hydration, time in nature, journaling, exercise, sleep. All these factors contribute to my overall health and peace-of-mind, but how can I do it all?

Last summer, I endured a terrifying situation where a man was determined to break into my home, and he was very persistent. This rattled me to the core and felt like something I really needed to recover from. In order to heal, I set out to increase all the possible ways of taking care of myself.

I wanted to nurture and nourish myself with loving kindness. So, I made lists, put everything in a calendar, shared with friends and clients, and proceeded to *try* to take good care of myself. But the checklists and goal-oriented mindset just stressed me out even more. I remember working at my desk and wanting to take a little break. I stood up, stretched my arms over my head, and said, "What can I do to take really good care of myself right now?" The "right now" was the key.

It felt like fun, rather than a task. It became a joy! I could have some water, take a walk, pet my dog, meditate for five minutes. There was always an immediate answer when I asked that question. So, I went from being someone who tries hard to take good care of myself, to someone who's eager to discover what good thing will I do for myself...*right now!*

I'll be fasting forever with these five important questions to steer me. And, perhaps in this sixth year, I'll learn the next important question. Stay curious, stay tuned!

I could *feel* it all along. From that third day in my mother's kitchen when I was overcome with feeling like myself for the first time in years, to the daily progress, restoring my health, being patient, and trusting my body.

But it's certainly useful to have external endorsement! Research demonstrates that daily fasting puts the body and brain into deep repair. The world's neurology and longevity experts, along with metabolism and hormone professionals, as well as gastroenterologists and cardiologists consistently confirm that we will feel better and live longer if we intermittently fast – eat in an eating window.

For me, the science coupled with my daily Intermittent Fasting practice was reinforced and celebrated a month ago in a very personal way. "Wow, you take really good care of yourself. Do you intermittent fast?," the doctor exclaimed as she pored over the battery of tests administered. "Your biological age is 40."

Unheard of. A 59-year-old menopausal woman who had nearly given up five short years ago, turned back the clock with a daily fasting regimen. For me, this gentle, natural practice is a sacred ritual. I won't mess with it. It has integrity to work *with* my body in this way. And I'm happy.

My heart is filled with gratitude for my dear Mom – for my life – from the beginning and for the next fifty years. Restoring my health all started with her generous listening, her prayers, and that first magical question, "How may I support you?" From her kitchen to mine, and now perhaps to yours, let's keep asking those curious, magical, uplifting questions.

Five Questions / Five Years

(Tear out this page and carry it with you. Ask yourself these five questions every day—multiple times per day as needed.)

1. When am I eating today?

2. Am I experiencing this "hunger" feeling because I'm sleep deprived, stressed, hurt, annoyed, bored, anxious, sad, avoiding something, or think I deserve a reward?

3. Given what I have going on for the next few hours, will I feel my best in a Fed or Fasted state?

4. What delicious food does my body need/want today?

5. What can I do to take really good care of myself right now?

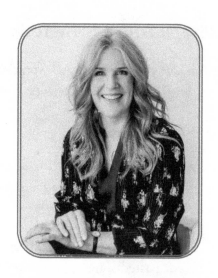

LAURIE LEWIS

Laurie Lewis lives in Portland, Oregon, with her snuggly pup, Violet. As a certified integrative health coach, she is enlivened by guiding thousands of people around the world to take very good care of themselves with Intermittent Fasting as the foundation. She can be found at Fast Forward Wellness, and her bestselling workbook *Celebrating Your Vibrant Future: Intermittent Fasting for Women 44 to Forever* will celebrate a re-release in June 2022.

Connect with Laurie here: https://fastforwardwellness.com

Chapter 3

FROM THE LOWEST OF LOWS

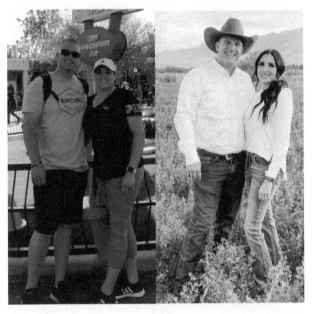

2018   2021

by Star McEuen

My story starts out like most, but first let's start with a bit of a back story. I always have felt like food has been an "issue," or something I would always think about. I thought I needed it at every special event. Everyone was always eating Breakfast, Lunch and Dinner, snacks, treats, etc. We would go out to eat to celebrate. We would eat when we were sad. We would eat just out of complete habit or because "it's time to eat." Not because we were truly hungry and listening to our own bodies. We most often than not quiet our own ghrelin hormone (the hormone that is produced in the stomach to let us know when we are hungry) because we are merely eating when we are "told" to by society, our boss, our parents, etc. No wonder our health journeys are so complicated; there is so much conflicting information out there, we don't even know what to do or who to believe or where to begin.

I was born in 1982 in Fountain Valley, California. Both of my parents were hippies and on the move. Shortly after my 1st birthday, we landed in a small town in Northern Arizona where we planted our roots. I am the only child and that is both a blessing and a curse. I had a rocky childhood, became diagnosed with Anorexia and Bulimia at age 13, and then what I believe saved my life was getting pregnant at 16 years old. I was 17 when I had my precious baby girl. After she was born, I never went back to my old habits of eating disorders. Instead, I got into the fitness world.

In 2002, I married my first husband and had 3 more beautiful girls in 2003, 2005, and 2007. During these years of having babies back-to-back, I would do all the "at home" DVD videos, go on daily walks with other mom friends, exercise around the park and even do our DVD workouts together sometimes to stay motivated. I was in my 20s and the weight just seemed to fall off after each baby.

The end of 2009, I met my forever soulmate and gained two bonus kids. We got married in April of 2010. Being in love, having a healthy and happy relationship, I put on a little weight. I got a little chubby for my liking, so by 2010 I was starting to search the web for, "How to lose weight quick," etc. I started with the meal replacement shakes and doing Zumba® at a local gym. I soon found my love and passion for dancing and became a Certified Zumba® Instructor and later went on to find a love for CrossFit®. I also went to school in 2013 to be a Certified Personal Trainer through the International Sports Science Association. I was extremely focused into fitness, working out and getting stronger. I loved seeing my progress, the muscles I was building, and for the first time in my life I was happy with the person I saw in the mirror. But that girl had to work very hard for what she had. I was in the gym for two to four hours a day, if not longer, doing strength training, then my CrossFit® workout, and either teaching Zumba® class or attending my best friends' Zumba® class. It was very time-consuming. But for this "season" in my life, it all worked for me. I can't remember how I was eating at the time, but it worked for me.

Then in August of 2015 we decided to build a home, which was extremely stressful and took a lot of my time. Getting to the gym was nearly impossible because other things took precedence. We were living with family friends while our house was being built and that alone made everyone and their schedules just off. We spent a lot of time driving and checking on the new house and it made it difficult to make home cooked meals and we would end up eating out because it was easier. This cycle repeated until our house was complete in November of 2015. This was about the time that my solid muscle body at about 160 pounds started to slowly pack on the weight. In 2016 we had some devasting news that changed our family dynamics and that's when the depression and the real weight gain started. I remember one day seeing the scale at 182 pounds and was looking in the mirror crying, asking myself, "How is this me?" Former personal trainer, Zumba® Instructor and fitness freak and now my weight is just going up and up. I felt so out of control, so confused, extremely depressed and fatigued all the time, everything hurt. This was all around the same time we were getting settled into our house and it was the start of a new year (2016) so I started trying everything to lose weight AGAIN. The meal replacement shakes, Phentermine (for a very short time), not eating (I was still spiking my insulin all day with something–protein shake, protein bar, bagel, oatmeal, a "low calorie beverage"), just taking bites here and there, but never really getting any nutrition.

Then I got to a point where I felt like I basically "gave up" because no matter how hard I tried, the weight just kept piling on. I remember seeing 199 pounds on the scale and I murmured to myself, "If I hit 200 pounds, I will kill myself"! YES, I said it, I KNOW it is awful to say and how sad is that. I remember just breaking down and crying because I felt so empty, I had completely lost myself and felt like a completely different person and I just couldn't understand why I couldn't lose the weight.

At this point, I thought my hormones have to be out of whack so I got those checked, I got put on thyroid medication and they swore I would feel better and get all my energy back and feel like myself again, etc. Well, that never happened. Then they did bloodwork and found I had high cholesterol, which was really no surprise, because my dad had quadruple bypass surgery at age 39, so I knew I was headed down that same horrible path if I didn't get ahold of this weight gain and start to lose weight. At this point, I was also prescribed Antidepressants (highest dose possible – 2 different ones) because when you are overweight, you feel terrible, you become a sad, miserable person and the doctor gives you medication for your symptoms. But they weren't addressing my "problem." My symptoms were real, my pain was real, my misery was real, my weight gain was real, the doctors were trying to help but we couldn't find the underlying cause. I avoided pictures, I was always hiding behind someone if you found me in one, and I became a complete recluse from everything and everyone. I was not myself for a good 4+ years, which makes me incredibly sad as a mom and wife because I feel like I lost out on some good years.

On May 9, 2019, I weighed in 30 pounds heavier than when I was 9 months pregnant, I was 207 pounds, my last recorded weight. At this point I was beyond ready to give up, the doctors weren't helping, I still felt miserable, and my bloodwork was showing no improvements. Then on July 22, 2019, I got a text from an old high school best friend, and she sent a picture along with it. I couldn't believe my eyes. She looked just as she did in High School, not only so thin and absolutely gorgeous, but young, her skin looked the same, she really looked JUST like she did back then. I quickly replied with, "You look amazing. What have you been doing?" Her reply, "Aww thanks, you should try Intermittent Fasting, I've been doing one meal a day for two years now, I'm the same size I was in college and I feel better than I ever have. Star, I know you hate to read, so get the book on Audible®. It's called *Delay, Don't Deny* by Gin Stephens. It's worked wonders for lots of people I know."

It took me a few weeks to download the book, but as soon as I did, I just cried listening to it because I just KNEW this was my answer. While I was listening to the book so many things would pop in my head and I was like, "I can do this; I don't even care for breakfast foods." Then I got to the part in the book about the clean fast and I was like wait, NO gum, no diet soda, no coffee with my beloved Stevia and creamer, no breath mints, no sugar free candy, no zero calorie energy drinks, no lemon in my water. I felt like the list went on and on. I will admit, it was all a huge shock to me, too, because our entire lives we are told the complete opposite, so WHY should I listen to this lady? Well, her story sounded a lot like my story, we'd been down every "diet rabbit hole" and always found ourselves feeling defeated and back at square one, with usually some more weight gain. At this point I had tried literally everything to lose weight and for some reason at this stage in my life all those "old things" (the gym, counting macros, weighing my food, meal replacement shakes) were NOT working and I was completely exhausted with ideas. For some reason Intermittent Fasting sounded simple and easy and like it didn't take much effort. There was no "diet plan" I had to follow, no calorie counting, no macros, no meal prep, no points, all I had to do was just clean fast and then I could feast and fuel my body in an appropriate eating window. It seemed so doable, and I was desperate.

On August 19, 2019, I started IF with a true clean fast, meaning I only had plain water (no lemon, no zero calorie flavors, no cucumber, strawberries, etc.), black coffee (not flavored beans, ground up and brewed, this is not a clean fast because the beans were flavored), black tea (be sure to always read labels because they are sneaky and add stuff–if it says citric acid, that will break your fast–tea leaves and water only on the label), or black green tea (freshly brewed with a tea bag and water is best).

I also started with OMAD (one meal a day). In Gin's book *Delay, Don't Deny*, she started with OMAD and about a 5-hour eating window so that was my goal. I was so tired of feeling crappy and being obese and I just wanted to feel better as fast as possible. For more information on Clean Fasting and OMAD, please refer to Gin's new book, *Fast. Feast. Repeat.*

In the beginning, I wasn't aware there were apps to help you log all your information, so I did it all in my notes on my phone. I would log what time I opened my eating window and what time I closed. Every day I would wake up, use the restroom, take my clothes off and jump on the scale, that way I would have an accurate number each day for my weight. Then at the end of the week, I would add up each day's weight, and divide it by seven days to get my daily average. This is the only way to get an accurate scale weight. Beware: the scale lies and does not measure our true progress and success. I have learned now that there are two apps available that are wonderful and will do all this math for you: (1) The Window App tracks your fasted hours, eating window length, along with the time you opened and closed (all very important on your journey) and (2) The Happy Scale app is a great app as well. You put your weight in daily and it will average it and show you your downward trend. If at all possible, I do discourage the scale with my IF clients. When we start Intermittent Fasting, we need to understand and commit to fasting for the long haul because we will never stop fasting no matter what that scale says; we will always fast for our health and wellness. I also logged my food in my notes and over time this tool really helped me to identify what foods I was really eating and how they made me feel. When you are only eating in a small time period, you are able to pinpoint the foods better that might be affecting the way you feel.

Back then I had a part-time job and got home around 1 or 2 in the afternoon, so I told myself to get up, get ready, get the kids to school, grab your water and off to work. I was always an all cream, with a splash of coffee kinda girl, so when I read I had to have black coffee, I boycotted it and decided water only. I felt so good, and the scale was moving and all I was doing was waiting to eat, it almost felt natural. I would usually break my fast with a snack of whatever sounded good, then later I would eat dinner and close. Over time, that got easier and I really liked eating dinner with my family so I would try to push my eating window until 4p.m. or so. Every month I felt better, my body was hurting less, my mental clarity was amazing, I was finally starting to feel like myself again. When I was about a year into fasting, I felt like I started "binging," getting hungry earlier than normal. I was eating two plus meals a day when for over a year I was strictly OMAD, I couldn't figure out what was happening. I reached out to a few fasting expert friends of mine and I soon figured out, after deliberating, what was happening. I was so hungry when I opened my eating window I would eat a large "snack," then I wouldn't eat dinner and then fill up with a sweet treat. I was getting no protein, no nutrients; therefore, I was not staying satisfied, and the food I was consuming was not sustaining me through the next day. I was getting hungrier earlier and felt like I needed more than one meal because my body was trying to catch up on nutrients. After I figured out I needed to break my fast with my main meal, fasting got much easier, soon getting to 20+ hours was no problem. Gin always says, "tweak it till it's easy" and sometimes you have to move your hours around and find what works best for you in the moment. Remember, you can't "mess up anything" because each day is a new day to do better.

One thing I did as I reached maintenance was focused on getting to 20+ hours fasted every day with an eating window of one to three hours. I try to break my fast with my main meal. Some days it works and some it doesn't and that's okay, too. That's life. I try to get to 20 hours fasted, but some days I can barely get to 16 or even 15 hours fasted, but for the majority of the time, I feel best when I get to 20+ hours. My eating window will vary from day to day. I really try to listen to my body and eat for my goal as much as I can. I'm a very busy mom of 6 children, so things don't always "work out" as planned, in my head, but I try my best daily to eat for my health goal and to really truly listen to my body.

Bloodwork doesn't lie. In 2014 when I was at my "healthiest," with extreme diet and exercise, my Cholesterol total was 208, Triglycerides 71, HDL 60, LDL 134, T3 117.

In 2017 my Cholesterol total was 314, Triglycerides 124, HDL 60, LDL 245, and my TSH 5.8.

In November of 2019, 3 months into IF, my Cholesterol total was 209, Triglycerides 100, HDL 43, LDL 145, and my TSH 0.097.

In 2020, with no exercise and only Intermittent Fasting, my total was Cholesterol 209, Triglycerides 58, HDL 54, LDL 144 and my TSH 3.17 (working on its own now).

Fasting has been the easiest thing I have ever done for my health, wellness, and weight management. After six months of IF, I was able to get off all antidepressants and my thyroid medication. After walking many health paths in my 40 years of life, this is the first time I feel good, have natural energy, awesome mental clarity, and I have maintained my weight loss of 81 pounds for over two years now. I don't have to worry if my jeans or swimsuit will fit when the time comes. For the first time in my life, I know how to maintain a healthy weight and that gives me unbelievable freedom. Whether you have weight to lose or not, I believe everyone should be an intermittent faster for the health benefits alone.

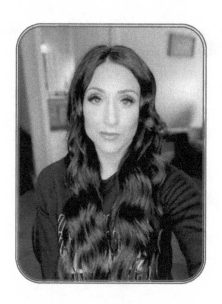

STAR MCEUEN

Star McEuen lives in Pima, Arizona. She and her husband are business owners of a small window coverings company, they share 6 children, with 4 busy high schoolers left at home. Star loves to cook and bake homemade meals and treats for her family. Star has been a stay-at-home mom, Massage Therapist, Zumba® Instructor, Personal Trainer, and is now a daily IF Accountability Coach. She is caring and sympathetic to others' needs, has a passion for health and fitness and helping others achieve their optimal health, through Intermittent fasting.

Connect with Star here: www.lovemyifinglife.com.

Chapter 4

GETTING OFF THE ROLLER COASTER RIDE FROM MORBID OBESITY TO FREEDOM – AN INTERMITTENT FASTING TALE

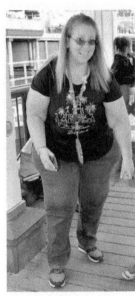
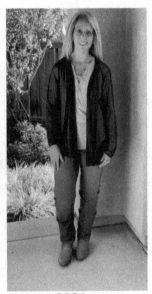

2019 2021

by Allison Woods

Intermittent Fasting changed my life! I've lost a significant amount of weight and gained more than I ever could have imagined, all without dieting, counting anything other than time, and eating delicious foods I love. Since finding Intermittent Fasting in May 2019, I have released over 140 pounds and have experienced well over 100 Non-Scale Victories (NSVs).

That's where I am now. That's not where I've spent most of my life.

So let me tell you how my rollercoaster ride with dieting and weight loss began.

I have been morbidly obese for as long as I can remember. My first diet was when I was nine years old. I was taking tap and jazz dancing lessons and was having difficulty doing all the footwork. I knew I was the biggest one in the class, and I was miserable. I begged my mom to help me. She had me do the same diet she was on at the time. It was awful, fake chocolate shakes and "candy bars" that were more like Styrofoam® than anything else. Did it work? I doubt it. I don't remember feeling much better at dancing class or being smaller.

In my early 20s I became a drug addict, primarily because I loved that it took away my appetite. I wound up in rehab at age 24. It was there that I was introduced to Overeaters Anonymous®. While staying abstinent from drugs and alcohol became part of who I am (I've been sober since June 9, 1993), staying abstinent from binge foods continued to be a struggle.

Over the next 30+ years I tried all kinds of diets, weight loss centers, schemes, and gyms, all to try to control my weight. I've tried Jenny Craig®, Nutrisystem®, Diet Center®, liquid diets, cleanses, Weight Watchers® multiple times, counting calories, macros, and carbs, among others.

Through all my efforts, I never got below the obese category. Interestingly, I couldn't even say the word obese to describe myself until very recently. It hurt too much. I would say "I'm overweight" or "I'm big," but never obese.

By the time I was 42 years old I had dieted my way up to 369 pounds. I could not stop eating the foods I knew were making me miserable.

I felt completely stuck. I decided my only way out was to have gastric bypass surgery. I was determined to be successful. This tool was the one I needed!

Was I successful? Yes and no. Two years after my surgery, I had lost over 150 pounds. I felt really good. I was looking better than I ever had. I was wearing size 16 jeans and felt so happy with my progress. And then, the scale started going back up. My beautiful size 16 clothes started getting tight and moved to the back of the closet.

During this time, I met my wife, and we became engaged. I picked out my wedding dress when I was at my smallest size. By the time it arrived a few months later, it no longer fit. I was so desperate that I started trying everything I knew to get the scale to go back down. In the end, I needed to have the dress completely altered.

Soon after we married, I was pregnant with our son. By the time he was 4, I had regained over 70 pounds. I could lose about 20 pounds with one diet scheme or another, only to bounce back up a month or two later. I was now back to wearing sizes 20-24 as I rode the roller-coaster again.

I was starting to think this was the best I would ever be and tried to convince myself I was happy in this size. It didn't work, though. Deep down, I was miserable and had this overwhelming self-loathing. I was embarrassed. I felt ashamed. I was uncomfortable. I was scared. I could barely keep up with my son. It was really difficult to get down on the floor to play with him. It was even more difficult to get back up.

By this time, I weighed 284 pounds and my size 24 pants were getting tight.

Then, just before I turned 50, an acquaintance told my wife about Intermittent Fasting, and she was very excited for me to learn about it. I heard that you had to eat a certain way with Intermittent Fasting, primarily following a ketogenic diet. Considering that I don't really enjoy eating meat, and that potatoes, beans, and fruit are among my favorite foods, I knew I wasn't going to be able to follow that diet. I thought to myself, here's yet another diet that works great for everyone else but won't work for me.

However, the part about not eating for a period of time during the day seemed doable and it made sense to me. I'd never been a big breakfast eater and don't enjoy most "healthy" breakfast foods. Skipping breakfast seemed so natural.

I found some groups on Facebook® that said you could have some number of calories (I honestly can't remember how many) during the fast. So, diet drinks and chewing gum were ok during the fast. I started with 16:8, but really struggled. I couldn't do it consistently day after day. I was ravenous by the time my eating window opened. The scale was slowly creeping back down the same 20 pounds as the past four years. Yet, I didn't feel any of the benefits everyone raved about. Why??

The answer was clean fasting. Once I discovered Gin Stephens' book *Delay, Don't Deny*, I read it in one night. Everything in that book spoke to me. I *knew* I could do this.

I started clean fasting the next day. That was August 27, 2019. I have now been clean fasting for almost three years. I have more energy, less pain, less inflammation, and better health than I ever have. This is where my rollercoaster ride with dieting ended.

I feel GREAT! This is now my lifestyle and I love it!

During the first one-and-a-half years of Intermittent Fasting, I lost 120 pounds and turned my health issues around. My knees and shoulders stopped hurting, my plantar fasciitis disappeared, and my doctor gave me a clean bill of health.

When I started Intermittent Fasting, I ate everything. Over time, healthier, nutrient dense foods became more attractive. Ultra-processed foods were no longer window worthy. Most important to me, the constant food chatter in my brain quieted down.

And then it came back. I found myself snacking, lengthening windows, and shortening my fasts. At this point I was still in the "overweight" category on the BMI charts. Stuck there for months while my clothes started to get snug.

In May 2021, I was ready to take a deeper look at my food choices. I was going to bed with stomach aches and feeling too full, which interrupted my sleep. I was sad and unhappy more often than not. I was losing energy. Many non-scale victories were slipping away.

I decided I had had enough. I did some digging and read a lot. It seemed like everything I read at that time regarding how to stop overeating in my eating window talked about sugar and flour. I really didn't want to feel this way anymore. I was ready to listen to my body and make a change. I decided to take the *Delay, Don't Deny* mantra to heart and go sugar and flour free for one month. I also tightened up my eating window back to my four-hour sweet spot.

I felt better, my thinking was clear again, and I was no longer bingeing. At the end of the 30 days, I was feeling so good that I decided to continue with no sugar or flour in my eating window. Incredibly, I reversed the direction the scale had been heading and dropped another 25 pounds. I was (and still am) in the "normal" range on the BMI scale for the first time in my adult life! This is more than I ever could have imagined. Never in my life did I believe I would weigh in the 140s. I didn't even think my body was capable.

I'm so excited about how much freedom I've gained from Intermittent Fasting, I want to shout about it from the rooftop! I tell anyone who will listen about Intermittent Fasting. Now my wife, mom, many friends, and neighbors are all Intermittent Fasting and feeling better than they ever have.

Intermittent Fasting has given me more than just weight loss. It's given me the desire to be healthy! I never really cared about my health before and would avoid going to the doctor. I felt like why should I bother? I was overweight so nothing I did would really make a difference, would it? Now, I want to be the healthiest I can. I enjoy taking care of myself on a daily basis. I don't do it perfectly, but I do stay consistent.

Knowing that I'm waking up each day no longer morbidly obese, no longer having pain in my knees, feet, and shoulders, knowing that I'm no longer putting my health at risk with high blood pressure, being pre-diabetic, insulin resistant, I can't think of anything better to celebrate!

So what have I gained by losing with Intermittent Fasting? More than I ever imagined was possible. I thought losing weight was just about how you looked in the mirror. Now I know the difference. I now have confidence in myself, my body, and my abilities. I really like who I am today and I'm no longer afraid to take risks and do things I think would be fun, like climbing a giant set of stairs at an amusement park to ride a slide with my son or taking a long hike through unfamiliar territory. I used to say no to these types of experiences because I *knew* my body couldn't handle them. I'd be too winded, in pain, or would not fit. I don't feel like that anymore and it's exhilarating!

I didn't realize just how cloudy my thinking was when I was eating all day. Now that I eat in an eating window, I'm no longer in a brain fog like I used to be.

I now have an off switch! Eating throughout the day, my hormones were out of whack. With Intermittent Fasting balancing my hormones, I finally recognize (and trust) when I've had enough to eat. I no longer need to eat for future hunger.

I'm still surprised by the increase in energy I've gained. I WANT to take the stairs, park farther away from the entrance, or run around with my 6-year-old. When he asks me to play with him, I don't hesitate to get down on the floor as I know I'll be able to get back up.

I also love going for walks now, which is something I always tried to convince myself I enjoyed in an effort to "move more and eat less." Now I actually want to go. I love dancing and currently take three dance classes, one of which is a performance class. I didn't have the stamina and confidence for this prior to Intermittent Fasting.

The thing I love the most about Intermittent Fasting is that it's all up to me. I can hear what my body is telling me about the quality and quantity of foods it needs. Nobody is telling me what or how to eat. It's a flexible lifestyle that I can adjust if I want to accommodate special events, vacations, and holidays.

Now, at age 52, I'm the thinnest, healthiest, and happiest I have ever been. For the first time in my life, I'm maintaining a right-sized body. The best part is knowing I'm off the dieting roller coaster forever.

Intermittent Fasting has made all the difference!

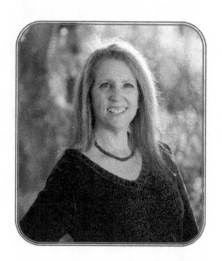

ALLISON WOODS

Allison Woods, Founder of Your I.F. Coach, has been Intermittent Fasting since May 2019. She has released over 140 pounds and logged over 100 Non-Scale Victories (NSVs)!

Having been morbidly obese for most of her life, Allison is on a mission to teach everyone how to unlock their body's potential, ditch the diet brain, and enjoy delicious food.

Allison holds a Masters Degree in Public Health (MPH) specializing in Health Education, and a Doctorate of Psychology (PsyD) in Organization Development. She is an Organization Development Consultant and has many years of experience in health education and training, individual and executive coaching, facilitating groups, and career counseling.

In 2021, Allison combined her passion for Intermittent Fasting with more than 25 years of health education and coaching experience and went back to school and became a Certified Health Coach. She then launched her coaching business: Your I.F. Coach (www.YourIFCoach.

com). Allison teaches, guides, and supports her clients to no longer feel stuck and hopeless when it comes to their health goals. She wants to help everyone discover the freedom that comes with Intermittent Fasting to live a vibrant and healthy life.

Allison lives in Sacramento, California, with her wife Lana, their very active 6-year-old son, and three dogs. With her newfound energy from Intermittent Fasting, Allison enjoys bike riding, golfing, swimming, and dancing.

You can connect with Allison at www.YourIFCoach.com.

Chapter 5

A HEALTHY FOUNDATION

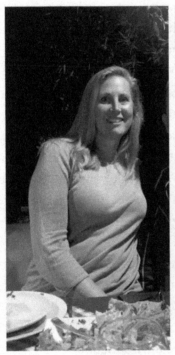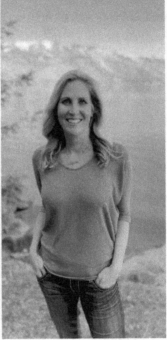

by Beth Wray

In construction, a solid foundation is essential. A strong foundation keeps a structure standing even when the forces of nature wreak havoc around it. The same is true for our bodies. They hold up best when they are healthy and well cared for. This is great news in relation to Intermittent Fasting (IF)! We are all born with a solid foundation of IF. Babies fast when they sleep and don't have the ability to break that fast until food is provided to them. Healthy babies are born with the correct hormone balance allowing them to be fully in tune with their hunger and satiety signals. Babies cry to alert us when they need food. When they are no longer hungry, they naturally turn from the breast or bottle, refusing more food. Essentially, everyone is born an intermittent faster. Then life gets in the way. As we age, societal and cultural influences affect our relationship with food, as do our emotions and our learned coping mechanisms. This is where things can get messy.

Many of us begin eating for emotional reasons rather than simply for physical nourishment. We eat to self-soothe, to numb, to fill a void, or even to celebrate. I did that for many years; for long enough that my natural hunger and satiety hormones got out of balance. Sometimes I would go days without ever really feeling hungry. I would just eat when the clock said it was time for breakfast, lunch, or dinner. I'd snack out of habit or boredom between meals and while watching tv. Other days, I would feel ravenous even though I had recently eaten a large meal. How could I possibly still be hungry?! At those times, as a response to my perceived 'hunger,' I reached for the addictive, highly palatable "convenience" foods – the ones specifically designed by the food industry to keep you craving more. Intermittent fasting helped me give up these habits.

At the age of 8, I began swimming, and loved the sport! It built my self-confidence and gave me a healthy outlet on which to focus my childhood energy. It also allowed me to eat copious amounts of food without gaining an ounce of fat. Nonetheless, I still fell prey to societal standards of the ideal body image. Instead of celebrating my strong swimmer's thighs, I became self-conscious and believed I needed to diet. Thus began many years of diet mentality, striving to be "perfect," and to achieve an unrealistic standard. It was a long battle that I was destined to fail; one that caused residual damage to my self-confidence along the way.

Growing up in the 1970s/1980s, calorie counting was the rage. I was taught to limit my calories and eat "low fat." Vegetables were basically non-existent in my diet, and I had a huge sweet tooth. When I stopped competitive swimming in college, I put on a few extra pounds, but kept the weight at bay through lots of aerobics classes. Then I got married and we started our family. With each of our 3 boys, I gained 30 pounds during pregnancy, but lost only 20 after each birth. Ultimately, this resulted in a net gain of around 30 pounds, which I struggled with over the next 20+ years. Every few years, I would get disgusted with myself and through willpower, exercise and diligent calorie restriction, I'd lose some weight. Ultimately, though, I was unable to sustain the lifestyle. Trying to limit my calorie intake by eating small meals throughout the day left me always feeling hungry and never feeling satisfied. It was a constant struggle for a self-confessed 'volume eater' like me. The yo-yo dieting took a toll on my self-confidence, and the amount of exercise required to maintain my weight took a toll on my body. If I got injured and was unable to exercise, the pounds would quickly pile back on. I was successful in most other aspects of my life, but was ashamed and embarrassed that I couldn't get a handle on my weight. It made me uncomfortable in social situations and lowered my self-esteem. That shame worsened my relationship with food and each weight loss attempt became more difficult. I often felt overwhelmed as a mother of three growing boys (I don't enjoy cooking), so I relied heavily on processed and ready-made convenience foods. Somewhere along the line, I began using food as my go-to coping mechanism for all of my feelings. Sad, frustrated, or bored? Food would comfort me. Special occasions and celebrations? Let's go out for drinks or celebrate over dinner! Food became the focus of my day. When would we eat next? What would I have? Maybe I shouldn't eat this "bad" food. If nobody sees me eat it, does it really count? It was a dysfunctional relationship and was not serving me well.

I felt like I had tried everything, within reason, to no avail. I may as well just accept myself as I was. After all, I was only about 30 to 40 pounds above the "ideal" weight for my height, and I was approaching menopause, so that wasn't so bad, right?! As much as I tried to accept that, I still felt uncomfortable in my own skin; like I was stuck inside the wrong body. One day I met with a friend who had recently lost weight and looked fantastic. Her skin glowed and she seemed happier and healthier than I had ever seen her. She introduced me to the concept of Intermittent Fasting. It sounded like the type of extreme "fad" diet that I wanted to avoid, but I listened with an open mind. She assured me that it was simple and that I could do it, too. There was no gimmick. I didn't need to buy special supplements and I could eat normal foods. It was a "lifestyle," not a "diet." She explained how 'breakfast' can be interpreted literally, as in "breaking fast," and it was not necessary to eat first thing upon waking. I learned more about the "clean" fast's ability to reduce circulating insulin levels, and it made sense to me as a mother of a son with type 1 diabetes. There was actual science behind this. Best of all, IF was free! I decided I'd give it a try. What did I have to lose?

At first, I could barely go without food for 14 hours (during most of which I was asleep). It was a challenge, but I told myself I could have whatever I wanted…later. On the days that I felt strong, I challenged myself to see how long I could go before opening my eating window. Some days were better than others and I learned not to panic when I had an occasional day that wasn't so good. I held myself accountable and did the best I could on any given day. If I was really craving something, even ice cream, I'd allow it as soon as my eating window opened. Sometimes I did exactly that, but other times I realized that I no longer wanted that particular food by then. It had lost its appeal. I was empowered by my fast and didn't want to undermine my own efforts. I began choosing more nutritious, whole foods within my eating window and filling up on those foods first. My motto became "hunger is not an emergency," and I started paying attention to what foods made my fasts more difficult (hint: sugar, alcohol, and processed foods). Knowing that certain foods cause me to be hungrier later makes it easier to say "no thank you" to them more often. It doesn't mean I always avoid them, because no foods are off limits to me. On the occasions when I do choose to indulge now, I thoroughly enjoy it, without guilt.

As a very "imperfect perfectionist," I have always been hardest on myself and carry the shame of not being able to live up to my own high standards. I am learning to give myself grace and self-compassion, and that the goal is "progress, not perfection." Brené Brown says that shame thrives in secrecy, silence, and judgment. I found an invaluable IF support system through Gin Stephens' *Delay, Don't Deny* community, where I connected with others who were just like me. I began sharing my story and experience with IF. Instead of feeling judged about my weight or my inability to lose it, I felt supported in my journey. The extra 35 pounds came off slowly and steadily in a way that seemed far easier than any previous attempt at weight loss. The accompanying body recomposition was amazing and the flexibility fit my life well. Along the way, I paid attention to patterns surrounding my food choices and hunger. My goal was to eat intuitively again, when I was physically hungry (not when I was emotionally hungry, and not based on a time on the clock).

Once the extra weight was off, I enrolled in the Institute for Integrative Nutrition (IIN) in an attempt to learn more and guarantee that I'd be able to maintain the weight loss. In many ways, I still viewed IF as a diet. It was difficult for me to reconcile how some people could seemingly eat all day and never gain weight, while others (who ate far less) struggled to even maintain their weight. IIN taught me about bio-individuality (what works for one person may not work for another). I also learned how our bodies store fat. After all these years of thinking that my body was working against me, I now understand that it was doing EXACTLY what it was designed to do. It was storing excess fuel in case I ever needed it (for a time of famine). Biological evolution hasn't kept up with technological evolution. Our bodies were not designed to be consuming food constantly. With innovations like refrigeration, convenience stores, and fast-food restaurants, our society now has food readily available at all times. People are used to instant gratification, and food is often used as a source of comfort.

I also learned how our bodies release fat. To let go of excess body fat, circulating insulin and glycogen stores both need to be low. Intermittent fasting helps to lower both of these (as does exercise and eating a low carbohydrate diet), which helps your body reach the desired state of ketosis. IF also provides the added benefit of increasing autophagy. Autophagy is the process of cellular self-cleaning and occurs the most during a fasted state. When our bodies are seldom in a fasted state, autophagy is reduced. Defects in autophagy are linked to various diseases such as neurodegeneration and cancer. So the added benefit of increased autophagy is enormous. Many people say they begin IF for the weight loss, but stick around for the health benefits.

Common misconceptions about IF are that it is difficult, overly restrictive, and that longer = better. None of these is necessarily true. On the contrary, most people find that, after an initial adjustment period, IF is simple and flexible.

I was born with a strong Intermittent Fasting foundation as a baby; eating when hungry, stopping when no longer hungry, and not eating if I wasn't hungry. These are the basics of intuitive eating. Somewhere in life, I lost touch with those. Beginning an intentional Intermittent Fasting practice as an adult allowed me to focus back on that foundation. The quiet of my fasts guided me to reconnect with my body, allowed my hormones to go back into balance, and gave me the opportunity to rebuild a healthier relationship with food. Through my education at IIN, I became certified as an Integrative Nutrition Health Coach and started my own business specializing in sustainable weight loss and emotional eating. Now, I have the opportunity of paying it forward by using my experience and education to support others in figuring out how to adopt an Intermittent Fasting lifestyle that suits them.

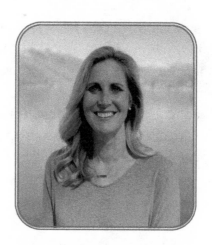

BETH WRAY

As a certified Integrative Nutrition Health & Wellness Coach, Beth Wray specializes in supporting those who struggle with their weight and want to find simple, healthy solutions for a sustainable lifestyle. Through private coaching, Beth works with clients to approach health holistically, and believes that good health is about far more than just the number on the scale or the food on our plates. She helps clients raise awareness surrounding their habits, identify patterns, deconstruct cravings, and incorporate simple changes in daily behaviors that add up over time.

Originally from the east coast of the United States, Beth now resides in the Pacific Northwest with her husband, Doug. Beth was a federal investigator before leaving the workforce to raise her family. Now the mother of 3 wonderful young men, in her spare time Beth enjoys playing tennis, hiking, and spending time with friends and family.

Connect with Beth at
www.simplehealthtransformations.com.

Chapter 6

AGING BACKWARD WITH DIABETES

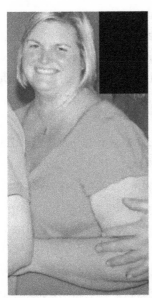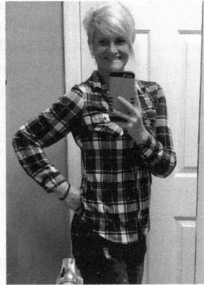

by Bethani Carter Johnson

I'm a 53-year-old grandmother with diabetes, high blood pressure, fibromyalgia, arthritis, and a poor immune system. I also used to be very obese, weighing 260 pounds at my heaviest. When I was eight years old, my parents divorced, turning my world upside down. My sister Melissa and I went to live with my dad and his parents after the separation. My grandparents loved us dearly, showering us with affection and junk food, all we could eat. I learned at an early age to suppress my feelings with food; food was comfort.

This unfortunate turn of events set me up for food addiction. Yep, there it is, I said it, I am addicted to food. The hardest thing about a food addiction versus a drug and/or alcohol addiction is that a living body can do without drugs or alcohol completely, but can't expect to survive long without a form of nutrition. Food is fuel, period!

Upon first beginning my journey, the end goal was to simply "reverse" my diabetes. I put the word "reverse" in quotations because I don't agree that anyone can ever actually "reverse." A person can become a diet-controlled diabetic, but will always be diabetic. This means that even after lowering A1C, this new WOE (way of eating) needs to continue for the rest of that person's lifetime. This is an entire lifestyle change, not a diet. Diabetics must learn how to have a brand-new relationship with food.

I was diagnosed with diabetes in 2010 and referred to a "diabetes counselor/nutritionist" for a series of classes on how to manage my disease. Now, let me preface this by saying, I am a registered nurse and SHOULD have been smart enough to do research on my own, but alas, I allowed someone else to manage MY body. I became a little suspicious of the class when the instructor told us to keep CANDY in case of a blood sugar drop! MY MOUTH DROPPED! Even back then I knew something wasn't right. I raised my hand and asked her to repeat herself and again she remarked that candy was the fastest way to raise blood sugar levels. Yep lady, you are correct; it will raise blood sugar– it will raise it to *dangerously HIGH levels*. Ugh, to think these people are "professionals." She also instructed me, at 260 pounds, to eat up to 180g of carbohydrates per day. Broken down, it would be 45g of carbs per meal with a 15g snack between each meal. They are teaching you that you need to eat every few hours to maintain your blood sugar. I have since learned that was wrong.

For the first few years after adopting the new "low carb" methods I had learned, I steadily began to lose weight. I was losing on average, 2 pounds a week. Of course, anyone will lose weight if they cut their regular intake of carbs in half. I was losing and feeling somewhat better, but I still had fibromyalgia pain, constant daily hip pain, and migraines out the wazoo. After losing about 75 pounds, the weight loss slowed down. I maintained and bounced between 180 and 200 pounds. By the time I was in my late 40s I began to slowly gain back my weight. This time it was mostly in my belly. That was new. I was puffier, my blood pressure was getting harder to control. I was taking two pills of one medication, plus another medication that had to be added later on by my Nurse Practitioner. My health was not improving, and my blood sugar/pressure wasn't in control at all.

It's February 29, 2020. Here I am, 51 years old, getting yearly labs done to get my metformin refilled (began that in 2010 when I was first diagnosed) and I find out that my A1C was 10.2! 10.2! I couldn't believe it! My head was spinning! I had been able to get off of my Victoza® a few years back and I thought I had a handle on things but, obviously, I was totally wrong. I know deep down it was the late-night snacking, Skittles®, SweeTarts®, chocolate, you name it and I would be grazing on it.

I felt so defeated. I had lost 75 pounds, gotten off Victoza®, and here I am with a high A1C. It just didn't make any sense. I asked my Nurse Practitioner what we do next, and she responded by increasing my metformin. I told her I couldn't take any more metformin because it made me constantly nauseous. She assured me she would call something in that I could tolerate, and I went on my merry way. When I got to the pharmacy, I was shocked to find that the new medicine she'd prescribed would cost $925.00 per month! At the time, we didn't have insurance, so I walked away wondering what in the world was I going to do? My stomach was in knots. How had I let myself get to this point?

How was I going to tackle this all alone? I felt so overwhelmed that I cried all the way home.

Facebook® isn't my favorite entity, but it does have its pluses, information being one of them. I had started following an Intermittent Fasting page my cousin Debbie had invited me to called Measure Me Life. I also started following a "reversing diabetes" group and, before I knew it, I was getting a lot of great info on fasting, low carb eating, and reversing diabetes. I love to do research, so I always navigate through the post comment sections and some of the time you can find very valuable information there. That method led me to Dr. Jason Fung. During the height of the Covid-19 pandemic, our Kentucky governor declared haircuts weren't "essential," so I found myself stuck at home for 10 weeks. During that time, I read three books by Dr. Fung. The first was *The Obesity Code*, followed by *The Diabetes Code*, and finally, *Life in the Fasting Lane*. Using those three books, along with a combination of Intermittent Fasting, low carb eating, strength, and determination, I saved my own life.

When I began, I would fast for 20 hours, and my morning fasting blood sugar would still be in the 190s! Imagine that?! It was a bit discouraging, but I kept hearing people say, "trust the process" so I hung in there and I'm really glad I did! I started with a 12-hour fast. Sounds easy, but I had no idea until I deliberately tried to make it 12 hours without eating. WOW! I thought I was going to die! Not really, a simple 12-hour fast goes like this: eat dinner at 5:30pm and nothing else before bed. If you wake up at 6am for work, when you wake up, you already had a 12-hour fast under your belt. It's really that easy! If you skip breakfast and eat at 12pm, you have just completed your first 18-hour fast. Another important thing to mention is WHAT you eat before fasting. I am able to fast for longer periods if I have eaten plenty of good fats and protein as my last meal. Carbohydrates are NOT essential to life; please try to remember that. We do not need carbs; we need protein and good fats.

There is something else you might hear often and that is becoming "fat adapted." The best way for me to explain that is when you eat a meal full of carbs, your body has to burn through them before it burns fat. For example, I eat 2MAD (two meals a day). I eat 10g of carbohydrates for each of those two meals and no snacks between or after meals. This has forced or trained my body to then burn the fat that I had gained over the years. If you eat a high carbohydrate meal, your body will burn through the carbs first and then if you follow up with a high carbohydrate meal you will only always burn carbs instead of fat. If you are not diabetic and simply want to lose or maintain your weight, a lot of people have success with Intermittent Fasting alone. However, if you want or need to lose a significant amount of weight, you will need to incorporate lower carb foods into your diet. Also, I do not count calories, only carbohydrates!

Early in the first year I found that my morning fasting blood sugar was very slowly starting to go down, but I was impatient and I wanted it to go down faster. To me it was a sign of my success, so I did a bit more research and found that the fastest way to get my morning fasting sugar to go down was by extended fasting. No matter how well my blood sugar ran throughout the day, my morning fasting sugar would remain high in the 160s. I started lengthening my fasts and to my surprise it worked! Once I had survived my first accidental 24-hour fast I tried again and I made it for 42 hours! I thought about my schedule and decided the easiest time to do that was from Sunday night at 6pm until Tuesday at 12pm. I am a hairdresser and work on Mondays, which keeps me busy, and also on Monday and Thursday nights I teach country line dancing, so I am literally busy all day on Monday. That made it SO EASY! I started to do a rolling 42–hour fast every other week and I did this for several months. In exactly one year my A1C went from 10.2 down to 5.8. I had lost 75 pounds, went from a size 14/16 to a size 4. The interesting part is that I NEVER had a weight loss goal. My only goal was to control my blood sugar with diet and get my A1C below 6. Following this new WOE had really paid off. Not only was I controlling my blood sugar with diet, but the weight was falling off! There were times when I would order a pair of jeans from an online consignment and by the time they reached me, they were too big. I never dreamed this would even work for me, but it was working and it worked quite well!

My husband and children immediately saw a difference in me. Not only in my weight loss, but my overall outlook on life! My depression was disappearing, I had much more energy, and I was just a happier person. My family has really supported me. Without their love and support I couldn't have been as successful. My husband David even changed his WOE to mine, and he has lost weight and feels better, too! In fact, I have so many people to thank, my beautiful mom Lyn, who taught me to never give up (she passed away recently), and my dad Don and bonus mom Sandy who has been encouraging me to write a book of my own.

Being invited to share my story in this book has been very empowering! I plan to write a recipe book of my own in the near future and share all that I have learned over the past few years including all the recipes I have created. I recently celebrated my 2-year anniversary of this new WOE and I feel AMAZING! I haven't had this much energy since I was a teenager. The pain from the fibromyalgia is gone and the only thing left to manage is my arthritis. I hope my story will encourage you to become your own advocate. Remember to research, read books, follow those who have had success and we can start AGING BACKWARD together!

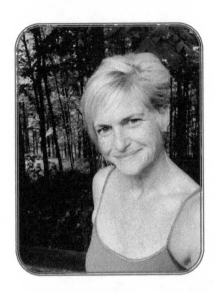

BETHANI CARTER JOHNSON

Bethani Carter Johnson is a mother of 2 and grandmother of 4 who was diagnosed with diabetes in 2010. Her passions are cooking, baking, and teaching line dancing in her community. She also loves to hike, kayak and take rides with her husband on his motorcycle. Her chapter describes a small piece of her journey, how she's improved her overall health, was able to stop diabetes medication completely, and get her blood pressure under control all with dietary changes and Intermittent Fasting.

Chapter 7

GRATEFUL HEART

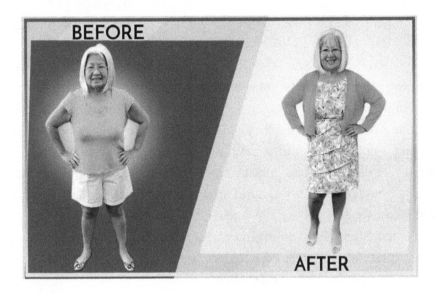

BEFORE

AFTER

by Carol Sakamoto

Most of my life has been spent watching my weight even when I was thin; it's become a part of me. In my early 20s I got pretty sick and was diagnosed with Hypoglycemia and Mononucleosis. It required me to give up carbs and sugar. I was already thin, but probably made me thinner due to the change in my diet. Before Intermittent Fasting, I was diagnosed with Acid Reflux, Gerd, and, in 2007, I developed a Schatzki Ring. That resulted in the narrowing of my Esophagus, which required that I be sedated and have my Esophagus dilated because I would find myself choking on food and it was hard to swallow. Needless to say, it was quite painful.

Our Cardiologist, Dr. Cesar Molina, M.D., FACC of Mountain View, California, along with our personal Crossfit® Trainer, Trac Nguyen, both suggested I try Intermittent Fasting. It was Jenny Hersenbach in a private Facebook® Group for silver haired ladies who told me about Gin Stephens' Intermittent Fasting program. I purchased Gin Stephens' book *Delay, Don't Deny* to learn about her Intermittent Fasting program. In addition to Gin's first book, I also purchased her second book *Fast. Feast. Repeat.* I read both books, listened to some Podcasts, and immediately started the program.

For several years, prior to Easter, our Pastor has been teaching us to fast one meal a day or what they call "Turn the Plate Over" for one meal. Fasting is not foreign or uncommon to me. Basically, we all learn to fast when we need to prepare for our blood to be drawn at lab, the typical fasting hours of 12:12. I was familiar with fasting from a spiritual sense, and I read about it in the Bible where God had fasted for 40 Days.

When I first heard about Intermittent Fasting, it wasn't too much of a surprise since I had learned to eat earlier in the day due to my Gerd issues where it was best to eat earlier to allow food to digest before bedtime, to alleviate the heartburn, and problems with acid reflux that are associated with this issue.

I started Intermittent Fasting on May 27, 2020, at 157.2 pounds, which is a lot of weight for my 5-foot frame. I also work out three times per week doing Crossfit® and have been doing this it 11 1/2 years, so I'm accustomed to working out and being active.

I have always worked out in a fasted state, so this part was not hard at all for me. I read in Gin's book it's really good for our Human Growth Hormone as well.

I wasn't sure what to expect when I started Intermittent Fasting, other than I needed to shed some weight and lower my A1C. The surprise came when back in February 2021 my husband took a photo of me for Chinese New Year, and I saw my dinosaur collar bones emerging which I haven't seen in the past 40 years or so. Seeing is believing, so I knew even though the scales haven't budged much in the way I was expecting a lot was going on in my body. In reading Gin's books, I learned about Autophagy, the body's way of cleaning out damaged cells in order to regenerate newer, healthier cells. "Auto" means self and "phagy" means eat. In essence, the literal meaning of Autophagy is "self-eating." It is recycling and cleaning at the same time, just like hitting a reset button to your body. Even though our scales may never budge or move doesn't mean that Intermittent Fasting is not doing its job or working for us. In Gin's Facebook® group, we call this NSV= Non-Scale Victory. We are reaching and accomplishing goals without it showing up visibly on our weight scales.

Intermittent Fasting has made me healthier. As a result, my Schatzi's Ring, which was diagnosed back on March 1, 2007, has healed itself according to my last endoscopy back in October 2021. My doctor said there is no findings of the Schatzki's Ring. I know for a fact this is attributed to the Autophagy for the past few years; it healed itself. This is a miracle from God. No way did I ever feel or expect to be healed from this as there currently is no cure for this diagnosis. Praising God for His healing over my body.

On a typical day, my average Intermittent Fasting Window is 18:6, sometimes I have longer windows that extend over 20 hours, depending on how busy I am or if I am out running errands. I have also done longer fasts of 40 hours. In order to better understand how my body functions and what foods trigger insulin to spike, I have now started to monitor my blood glucose at home. It is not a requirement or a necessity, but more on the basis of wanting to better understand what triggers I have when I eat certain foods. Also, it helps me understand how long it takes for my Blood Glucose to return to normal after eating a meal.

In addition to my morning weigh-in on my Renpho scale, I decided to take charge of my health, and incorporated checking my blood pressure every morning, in addition to my morning blood glucose. I keep a daily journal to track my ups and downs. I've always known that I am insulin resistant, but by monitoring it, I am now more educated on how my body functions and works.

Intermittent Fasting has taught me that I really don't need to eat when I'm not hungry. As a child, we may not have been hungry, but that "lunch time" bell triggered us to eat because our school schedule revolved around our daily curriculum. I have learned that I may not be hungry for breakfast in the early morning and by checking my blood glucose if it is high, then it confirms that I am not hungry yet and need to wait until the blood glucose drops.

In the past year, I feel that I was squeezing in lunch even though I barely had breakfast, but was concerned about closing my window with only one meal, but maybe on some days it's what my body needs is only one meal. I never feel faint or lightheaded, so I know I'm on the right track if I eat only when I'm hungry. Intermittent Fasting is very easy for me due to no more counting carbs, calories, or weighing of foods. That was the diet brain mentality that I grew up with during my young adult years. Now I'm free and no longer follow that pattern.

When I reflect back on Weight Watchers® back in the 1980s, it was very controlling, daunting coming home with a scale, and weighing my foods. Then to log or cross it off from a chart that I had posted to my fridge door. Also, to check off the glasses of water I drank per day. I only did it a few times, but felt it was too time-consuming and having to think of each and every step to be successful in planning, shopping for meals, the time away from my family responsibilities to attend these meetings, in addition to the weekly cost. Whatever I lost would spring me forward and over my starting weight, so it had a negative effect on me.

Intermittent Fasting is basically free, no membership dues, just purchase books or join some private Facebook® groups for support, encouragement and advice. I have the freedom to enjoy my vacations, special occasions, without having to worry about calories or the type of foods I am eating and drinking. When I return home, I give myself a week to reset my body. At times, I have been known to do a kidney cleanse with coriander and water. Reminded me of growing up as a child, my mother would periodically make a watercress soup and feed it to us to help us to detox and get rid of toxins in our bodies.

It was on January 20th, 2022, that I decided to tweak and add more to my daily routine, to gain more control, become more knowledgeable about how my body functions. Because I am so cognizant about my hemoglobin A1C, I wanted to learn more about Intermittent Fasting and my blood glucose. I joined a Facebook® group and was introduced to Kattie Muir who has been walking alongside and coaching me. I have increased my knowledge and gained some great tips from her to incorporate into my daily life. I have lost an additional 5 pounds and attribute it to her coaching, encouragement and support.

In closing, I am grateful and thankful to my cardiologist, personal trainer for suggesting Intermittent Fasting so that I can live a healthier life at the most optimum weight for my age and body. The scale does not tell the truth of what is actually going on inside our bodies where there is an accumulation of inflammation, damaged cells from years of dieting, etc. Trust the process, as our scales do not reflect if our A1C is improving and in my case the miracle of my Schatzki Ring being healed as currently there is no cure for this ailment. Intermittent Fasting is great with a side benefit of weight loss.

My motto is "put on blinders like a racehorse, focus on your own fasting lane, and do not compare your journey to the next person, for each of our bodies are created uniquely and different from one another."

Our health is an investment, not an expense. If you don't make time for your wellness, you will be forced to make time for your illness. Our mental health and livelihood are the golden key in our senior years, so we can enjoy all that God has for us.

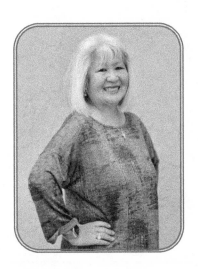

CAROL SAKAMOTO

Carol Sakamoto was born and raised in Palo Alto and Cupertino, California. She is of Chinese heritage and can speak some Cantonese. She resides in the heart of Silicon Valley with her husband of over 45 years, where they raised their 2 children, and are both now happily retired. In her working years, Carol had a career in Finance with various high-tech companies and her role was in Credit Management.

Carol and her husband enjoy gardening outdoors in their community plot harvesting organic produce, attending classic car shows and traveling together, when possible. Her goals and inspiration are to stay healthy, to serve her church and others where Jesus leads and guides her. Carol is grateful and thankful every day to our Lord.

Chapter 8

FINDING MY FOOD FREEDOM

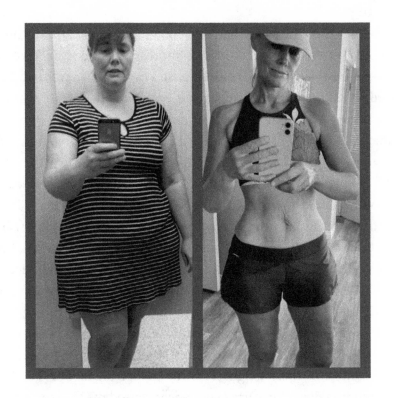

by Emily Harveaux

Beautiful soul reading this piece, do you long to feel free? Are you weary? Have you spent decades punishing yourself and your body with extreme weight loss efforts? Have you felt it was all your fault? Do you feel hopeless?

I know I did.

I am on the other side of a transformation. I am content, confident, whole, and healed. My body has followed this healing path and has established itself in a strong, lean form and a healthy size. This is how I got here, my story of how I achieved beautiful acceptance of my body and my whole self.

My Story

"Watch the greasy food with her," the doctor said to my mother during a routine doctor's office visit. I was mortified to be spoken of and judged under this doctor's critical eye, at a mere eight years old. I had noticed I was larger than many of my friends, but I had never heard my size or fatness being publicly stated before. I said nothing, of course, but the embarrassment and shame I felt was heartbreaking. As a child, I really wasn't sure who believed in me or thought I was worth much.

My younger years were marked by chaos, abuse, and insecurity. There were some important figures who instilled confidence in me along the way and helped me feel that I mattered. Do you know how these stable and safe people showed their love to me? Attention, time, and of course—FOOD! Not just any food either. It was nutritionally poor, damaging comfort food like donuts, cookies, and cakes. Yummy as a kid, but damaging to my body and mind.

My well-intentioned, deeply loved family members were eating very unhealthy foods and treats. They were also trying to stay slim and in control of their weight with the grapefruit diet or TOPS® or other trending diets. My early experiences caused me to associate love and safety with unhealthy sugary and processed foods. A seed was planted in my outlook toward food and diet. This was the beginning of my food addiction to sweets, breads, and non-nutritive foods. I had learned to associate strong emotional connections and safety with sugar and carbs.

During my teenage years, I continued to practice damaging habits with food. I was managing to keep my weight controlled by being active in cheerleading. However, my nutrition was still terrible. I was living off of Diet Coke® and candy bars. I was hoping to land a boyfriend by keeping my size under control. I hoped all of the exercise from cheerleading would keep me trim. This was a fun time in my life socially, but my habits were worsening including unhealthy weight loss attempts, over-exercising, restriction, and yo-yo dieting.

My 20s, 30s, and early 40s were full of diets and programs to try to manage my weight. I just couldn't figure it out. On numerous occasions, I was up and down the scale from the 170s to the 290s. By the time I had my four children, my weight had gotten up to 300 pounds several times. There was no denying my weight was becoming a real health concern. I was having energy drains, shortness of breath, and severe anxiety and depression. Worst of all, I had lost hope that I could feel good and keep up with the pace of managing my large family.

In Fall of 2017, I hit my rock bottom on self-esteem as I was again hitting my top weight of 300 pounds. I was still me underneath all of the poor health, inflammation, and fat. I wanted to live a full life and be the best mom possible. I was 46, over-exercising at 300 pounds, and I ended up with a meniscus tear injury on my left knee. I had been taking tap dancing classes and doing HIIT® training. My meniscus tear landed me on the couch for most of my days. During this couch chapter, I was fortunate that a friend had pleaded with me to read *The Obesity Code* by Dr Jason Fung and *The Complete Guide to Fasting* by Jimmy Moore and Dr. Jason Fung. I learned to fast effectively and successfully. I finally had a big piece of my ultimate health solution figured out!

I feel so fortunate that I found the correct answers to my weight problems! My problem was not one of calories in versus calories out. My issue was hormonal, caused by overeating addictive processed foods! My first step into health freedom was through Intermittent Fasting.

I learned that fasting was completely safe and healthy for my body. I felt wonderful during my fasts. I used short daily fasts, extended fasts, and all different varieties of Intermittent Fasting schedules to lose weight. It was working well and I was feeling wonderful! I had gone from 300 pounds to the 180s and was feeling on top of the world!

From 2017-2020, I was fasting, eating keto and feeling wonderful, but I still had a problem. I was completely addicted to carbs, sugar, and sweet tasting keto treats. These harmful foods had such a strong grip on me. I wondered how I could finally free myself from sugar addiction and whether it was even possible. I knew how to fast by then, but I didn't know enough about nutrition and how to feast!

A good friend of mine who was a seasoned intermittent faster had tried the carnivore diet and shared her day-by-day experience in a private Facebook® group. I read about her experience and I eagerly studied each word. She had so much hope! Processed food and sugar no longer controlled her. This sounded so extreme. Could it possibly work for me? Could this be the answer to me finally dealing with sugar, sweetener, and keto-treat addiction? I had to try it!

The carnivore diet combined with Intermittent Fasting was the ultimate answer for me. I began eating this way January 2, 2021, and I have never looked back. I had only planned to do this for one month, but I felt so amazing eating no sugar and no processed foods that I just kept going! Eating my healthiest foods made me feel the best I have ever felt. It has become such a passion that I now spend my time teaching those who want to learn how to safely feast, fast, and eat in this manner!

It has been remarkable to see the physical changes my body has gone through combining fasting with my nutrient dense diet. My weight is now in the 140s to 150s. I am the lightest and healthiest I have ever been! My waist is the smallest it has ever been, down to 26 inches. I am fully energized, fit, strong, and lean. I love the energy I have every day. My nutrition fuels my life as a mom, partner, coach, and educator.

A main passion in my life is to talk about and celebrate the food freedom I now feel. I have zero cravings! I work long hours without hunger or food calling to me at all. I eat the most delicious, delightful food possible. I have clarity of mind, no brain fog, no depression. My sleep is deep and energizing. My skin is smooth and nourished. I have personal boundaries like never before.

What I've discovered is that Intermittent Fasting combined with my proper nutrition are powerful tools and have drastically reduced my inflammation. I was shocked to find out that my depressed brain was actually an inflamed brain. Once my systemic inflammation was gone, my brain was in a healthier state. From what I know now, it's clear that I was missing the proper nutrition for my optimum mental health.

I had to become bold to honor my own body's healthiest choices. With the constant social pressure to eat, I've had to get strong enough in my fasting practice to forgo food while others are eating. And that made me feel quite accomplished, especially compared to how I used to be with food. I feel empowered when I'm at a gathering where everyone is eating and I no longer have that need or desire for food to enjoy myself. I'm no longer saddled with the social pressure of eating. This is true empowerment. I often feel such inner strength and peace as I sip on sparkling water while friends are eating. Of course I am free to eat as well, but the difference today is that I am in control of myself and it is completely up to me to have the food or not. One of my favorite things about going against the flow is that it makes me feel strong! It is a bold statement when we decide to be completely devoted to our personal health. This takes making a decision to put health first and continue to follow up on your life-giving choices. When I began approaching the world with confidence to put myself first by Intermittent Fasting, I started making waves. I was honoring myself so deeply and confidently that I ended up feeling limitless and proud with a strong sense of self.

You can hear my passion for excellent nutrition and Intermittent Fasting. This is the best I've ever felt in my life! What I've found is that feasting is actually the most important part of the process. I fill my body up nutritionally to have efficient, doable fasting periods. Once I have feasted properly, my fasts become natural and enjoyable. I look forward to fasting days because I have mental clarity and pure energy and my mood is calm and positive during my fasts. I actually prefer to be in a fasted state. While I'm fasting, I am more focused on the task at hand. I have also come to prefer exercising in a fasted state. All of these wonderful fasting benefits have come my way because I have feasted properly when it is time to eat.

When I talk about fasting and feasting, I like to share the perspective of animals in the wild. They don't fret, plan, or control their food. They have many cycles of feasting and fasting (while lions can go for a week without eating, they've been known to go for up to a month with no food—as long as water is available). Just like lions, once we are properly nourished, our body will happily and naturally fast.

What I found works well for me to build up to extended fasts is to go for 22 hours fasted, followed by a 2-hour eating window. Next, build up to fasting for an entire day (including the night before and after)—yielding roughly a 36-hour fast. Finally, stretch that time to 42 hours. This 36- to 42-hour fasting cycle is commonly known as ADF—Alternate Day Fasting. I do repeating cycles of ADF, and I will flex around social events and various activities. If I have a period where I want to be particularly productive, I'll set it up so that I'm fasting at that time. On the other hand, if I'm dealing with significant stressors or social events, I'll adjust it to approach those events in a fed state. Feasting on good nutrition in my eating window is what sets me up for easier, more successful fasting. Learning to feast well has been a game changer.

The best part of feasting and fasting is the food freedom it's given me! This is the ultimate win. Food Freedom is marked by the following benefits: absolutely zero cravings, confidence in social and emotional situations, feeling in control, and self-love. I am at my best, physically, mentally, and emotionally, when feasting and fasting. This is how I've reached my ultimate goal and have achieved long-term food freedom successfully.

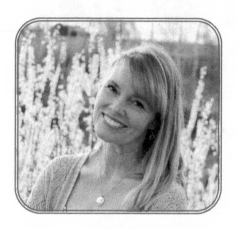

EMILY HARVEAUX

Emily Harveaux is a transformation addict who loves to inspire others on their journey to health and wholeness. She has released 150 pounds of fat from her body through feasting, fasting, and putting her nutrition first. She was at her heaviest weight at 300 pounds. She is currently in the 150s and feeling energized, motivated, and excited to show others the way to Food Freedom. She is married, mother of 4, Fasting and Carnivore Coach, and a co-host of The Butter Dish Gals Podcast. She teaches in a group coach setting and as an individual coach.

Connect with Emily at IG @melt.that.snow.

Email: EmilyHarveaux@gmail.com.

Chapter 9

FINDING COMFORT IN THIS LIFESTYLE

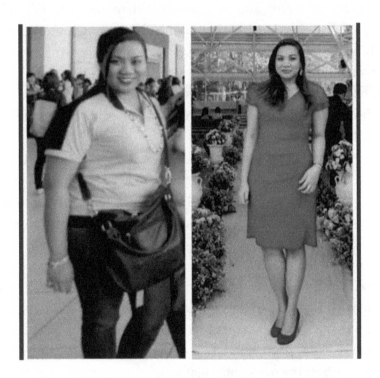

by Izzah Tiama Hemoo

Unlike most people, I didn't actively plan to start Intermittent Fasting. I just happened to accidentally be doing it, and when I realised there was something to this lifestyle I had accidentally embraced, I wanted to find out all I could about it and incorporate it into my life.

The truth of the matter is, I stumbled upon it at a point when I was stressed in all areas of my life, be it work or personal, and it became my saving grace.

I am what they call a third culture kid (maybe even fourth!), growing up in a different culture from what my parents were born in. I was born in the Philippines, but most of my formative years were spent in a beautiful little country in Asia called Brunei. I studied in Malaysia and Australia for university, and because of the strive for a good life, I have worked around the world, including the Philippines, a short phase in the US, and now am currently in the UK. But where will I be tomorrow? By the time this book is out, I may already be in another country. And I tell you this, because I want you to picture this nomadic Asian workaholic suddenly finding one constant in her life that made sense: Intermittent Fasting.

Taking a step back, turning to food for comfort was inevitable for me, as I had an immensely happy childhood, filled with love and, of course, food. It was and is our family love language, to celebrate occasions around a table filled with food. Eating together is what we love to do to this day.

Then the teen years came around and I thought I was a 'socially accepted' beauty because, plainly, my parents told me so. The world doesn't work that way. Quite quickly I found out I wasn't naturally beautiful in the socially accepted standards of the community I was in, being overweight, having glasses and the bane of teenage life – acne. And strange how the rose-tinted glasses of a loving family shielded me, as I only fully realised this when I was told to my face I was 'fat' by who I now see were cowardly bullies. I see where they are in life currently and I feel a sense of vindication that some at least know personally what being fat is. I speak about this calmly now, but doesn't everything feel so much more dramatic when you're young?

All grown up now, it feels odd to admit that the final act that veered me from thinking I was a beauty was being told as a teenager that that I looked 'exotic.' I was 12 and thought it was a compliment, but quickly found out the sniggering boys meant I looked like an entry from a safari. But these were the cruel ones. Life blessed me with my own social groups, without whom I would have ended up with much more hate in this world. So instead of focusing just on my looks, I was happy to find people who were my friends simply because I was me. I found other areas I could hone and shine in, did well in school, was active in school competitions and the like. I had my own interests and world, found the internet and dreamed, like most little bookworms, to write a book. I also have a memory of aiming to be a wine making nun (I blame movies!), so my high school self wasn't really one to rely on for my feasible dreams!

I hope you can see where I am going with this. While others worked on losing their fat, I decided I didn't care, something very alien in the 1990s where Kate Moss was the epitome of beauty (I was so happy when the J Lo and Beyonce eras came around!). Rather than lose the weight, I devoted myself to being 'busy' with school, friends, and interests, and this workaholism attitude which had protected me growing up from the pains of society also had me falsely accepting that my weight was something I could not change, so why should I? I should have tried, but thanks to my parents and friends, my self-confidence was largely drawn from something else inside me that told me I was worth more than just looks, which I believe we all are.

We are obviously worth more than our looks, but little did I know I was also building a bad mental attitude and unhealthy attitude towards food. That I could eat what I want since I was marginally successful in other ways. Fast forward to my adulthood where this attitude was carried over and I felt complete in my life despite my weight, but my one mistake was ignoring my health and always turning to food for comfort, and always looking forward to my next meal, whether I needed a meal or not.

As I aged, I gained weight slowly but steadily and while I hit a lot of my life milestones, including buying a house, car, getting my dream work and finding love with my now husband, I also hit my adult high of 240 pounds in my 20s and I am only 5 foot 4 inches. That was when my life finally changed health wise. Annual physical check-ups always told me the same thing, that I needed to lose weight; otherwise, my cholesterol levels and sugar levels were fine. But this particular year, the doctor was extra vicious and told me if I wanted to have children (which is presumptuous!) I needed to lose weight.

In the Philippines, its cultural to greet people with 'oh you have lost/gained weight' and years of my neglect to my physical self now meant that I was receiving the latter, that I laughed off. I was feeling it more though and was also wheezing going up the flight of stairs. My knees were acting up, I felt gout pains and I was quickly realising I would need to change my lifestyle if I didn't want to be less healthy than my 60-year-old parents.

Carrying over my busy lifestyle from my teen life, I had immersed myself in work and duties in my adult life. I was working side hustles as well as the IT world, and my 20s was a point in my life that I had jobs that had global teams working different time zones. Due to the time zone differences, we (not just me) would sometimes miss meals to accommodate a meeting. The rest were smart enough to eat and bring food to their workstation, but I was in one role where I was so overwhelmingly busy and yet having fun in the role, that I started missing my 5 meals a day routine. Shock of shock to my food addicted soul, I found out I didn't feel hungry and could be fueled by my one meal a day even when working 12-hour days. I was powered by black coffee and later realised

I was in ketosis while successfully working on projects delivery. It was a breakthrough for me: I could function without my food?

Looking back, I believe I turned to food for comfort out of habit. And finding out that food, which had always been my comfort, wasn't comforting anymore, I was reveling in not needing it as compulsively as I had once done.

And finally, Google® searches and social media and talking to friends led me to find out it was because I was not just simply 'skipping meals,' which sounds more criminal than it should be! I was unknowingly Intermittent Fasting. And it clicked in that moment for me to be curious enough to see what happened if I did it properly.

This isn't how I advocate finding out about Intermittent Fasting. Months of eating one meal a day accidentally led to me suddenly receiving greetings of 'Oh, you have lost weight' and compliments for a fat loss I wasn't aware was happening. I had been hiding that from people that I was skipping meals because missing meals isn't well embraced in Asia, and I was fully intending to return to my old lifestyle and wasn't actively working on weight loss and thought my one meal a day was heavy enough, and being a fact nerd, I needed to find out what was happening. I weighed myself, and though I was initially losing weight, somehow, I was maintaining a weight and not losing any more yet looking leaner. What was this magic and how could I be looking leaner with the scale staying the same?

It turned out it wasn't magic. Joining support groups online (especially Gin Stephens' Delay, Don't Deny: Intermittent Fasting Support Group on Facebook®) had me understand that by maintaining my OMAD (One Meal A Day) lifestyle (usually 20:4), it gave me body recomposition where I was maintaining my body weight, but I was losing fat and building muscle. There's a famous picture on the internet which shows that 5 pounds of muscle takes up less mass than 5 pounds of fat, so I don't rely on the scale, but I measure inches.

Weight loss is very much a mental shift of mindset as well and it took me a long time before I could start shopping for new clothes because I always felt that at any moment I would revert back to 240 pounds. I started incorporating exercise, simply because I could do the exercises now at a lower weight. The superficial side of me was reveling in the fact that at my peak weight of 140 pounds, I found clothes fitting better for the first time in my life and I could fit in sizes I last fit in when I was 15. And the best part was going back to that doctor for my next annual physical exam and her asking me how I lost the weight and teach her.

I hope this part resonates with others. I gained the weight back!

So, we have established that IF did work for me and I had reached my goal weight and was happy. As life would have it, I moved from my tropical country to the cold weather in the UK, and while I loved experiencing the UK, the change in temperature, being apart from my social circles, and being away from my husband and family, meant I went back to food for comfort and, of course, this quickly led to a swift weight gain, and I was back to almost 200 pounds. Needless to say, this was very disheartening as I felt I had ruined all the progress I had done.

However, my husband came over to the UK, and this was a huge help because he is a natural chef and he calmed me down. Together, we went back to an Intermittent Fasting lifestyle and I lost the weight again. When winter comes around, I now know that cold weather is a trigger, and I find it very hard to fast, but having a supportive husband who ensures our one meal a day is packed with nutrients and some treats, that makes it much easier!

Looking back at my Intermittent Fasting journey, it's had its highs and lows. But these days, I knowingly fast. In my 30s, it gives me a sense of peace and comfort knowing I no longer chase food, but plan meals to suit my lifestyle. I like that my clothes fit better and I can experiment. I do it for the health benefits, not just for weight loss and ultimately the time gain (you might be surprised how much time is spent eating). I have a better relationship with food these days, feel healthier and am working on getting to my peak healthy weight and maybe I'll even learn to cook! No matter where I am in this world, my husband and Intermittent Fasting will always be my constant.

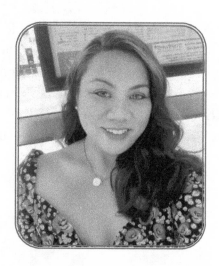

IZZAH TIAMA HEMOO

Izzah Tiama Hemoo is a Filipino married to a Mauritian and this means their food is a blend of both worlds. She works in IT, reads and watches tv for fun, and has always been a foodie.

These days, she eats consciously, experiments with fashion in her old age, and no longer runs to food for comfort. She enjoys reading and hopes to one day travel properly again.

As an avid traveler, Izzah is a Local Guide Level 5 on Google Maps®, enabling her to use her love of sharing photos of food and places for good by helping people who use Google Maps® and Reviews decide where to go and what to do in any part of the world.

Connect with Izzah on Instagram at https://www.instagram.com/treatsinmywindow/

Chapter 10

HOW I LOST OVER 100 POUNDS WITHOUT BECOMING LESS OF ME

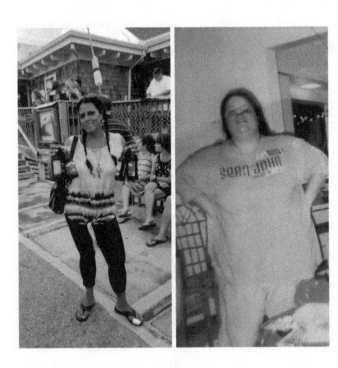

by Jackie Fitzwater

I lost over 100 pounds without losing all of my mind (I did "lose"/heal my "stinking thinking") and became more of me.

Enter Intermittent Fasting! Rather than eating my feelings, I "ate" my hunger, literally. Instead of numbing my emotions, I'd feel them and feel empowered by being hungry. I became ravenous for life, hungry for healing, and I followed the yearning hunger of taking my power back.

Enter dense nutrition and only putting into my mouth what I absolutely loved and/or what was healing. Though I was morbidly obese, I was "starving"/malnourished. A super food shake helped to provide nutrients and curb my appetite while fasting. I started using my hands for other creative pleasurable things (wink) instead of putting food into my mouth.

I weighed over 300 pounds; the scale stopped counting and so did I. I stopped counting calories while Intermittent Fasting and started counting the moments in life, little by little. For my ADHD brain, counting calories, carbohydrates, macros and micros, hey Macarena, would lead me to overwhelm and inaction or overreaction. Portion control color containers = 1 potato 2 potato 3 potato 4, so that was a green container, blue container, red light, green light, no go. The thought of the long shopping lists, money was extremely tight, and asking me to go to the grocery store was like asking an alcoholic to be a bartender = nope. I'd buy a few pounds of chicken (plus the other treats somehow jumped into my cart), cook it for weekly meal prep, then accidentally eat it all. Or I'd get too hungry before I cooked it and order a pizza or go through a FA(s)T food drive-through. Even if I was full, I'd keep eating because, duh, starving kids in Africa. Plus, the guilt and shame of "falling off the wagon" again would incite me to numbing it all with food. I had so far to go! I felt like I was going in circles, constantly setting myself up for failure. There had to be a better way!

Before Intermittent Fasting, after reading all about how vegans could walk on water (insert laugh), I tried to convince myself that I'd go to "hell" if I ate another piece of meat. Everyone knows that the cabbage soup diet was like holy water (face palm).

I started learning to work with myself instead of perpetually against myself. I slowly learned to go with the flow of Jackie instead of following the "prescriptions" meant for others. We are all different with unique desires, metabolisms, blood types, energy, nutritional needs, etc. I've never been a breakfast person, even though we hear that it's the most important meal of the day. I've actually never been hungry before a typical lunchtime. When I'd attempt to have a "healthy" breakfast, it only led me to devouring more calories that day. I'm always hungry at night, always, no matter what I've eaten or not throughout the day, and I'm ravenously hungry after an intense workout. Some "experts" say to exercise when you first get up, get it out of the way, and energize yourself for the day. That was another not fit Rx for me; I was exhausted and would sure enough consume significantly more calories! You know how many "experts" say don't eat after a certain time? That backfires for me every time (unless I'm doing an extended fast). Since I'm hungry later, that's where I typically keep my fasting window. I felt ashamed, like something was wrong with me. First, I had to understand that after enduring traumatic experiences as a child, it's sadly "normal" for people to become obese. I had to "get" that what happened to me was not my fault, while healing was my responsibility and within my power. I did the best I could with the knowledge I had. What once subconsciously made me feel I was keeping myself safe (coping mechanisms), then became my self-inflicted prison. I was coping the best I could, but/ and I yearned to thrive instead of simply survive.

My initial attempts at Intermittent Fasting, after not eating breakfast or lunch, I'd accidentally have several portions at a buffet or family size dinner. Oops! I added a shake to help curb my appetite and add dense nutrition. I was obese, yet nutritionally depleted, since I was lacking vitamins, minerals, and practically anything healthy! I love food that I love, like seriously, foodgasms are a thing! Instead of a buffet,

I'd pick that one thing I was craving and that, along with something healthy, would be worth me fasting for. I need a reward, something to motivate me! It could be a new buzzing bedroom accessory, since I'd recently discovered the benefits of self-pleasure, a new trip/experience, or a new restaurant. A certain sinfully scrumptious sub was sometimes my incentive. The whole thing was too many calories, so I'd cry a little inside while I gave half away. Sometimes I'd dump water on food so I wouldn't eat it. I'd think of the starving kids, since my family initiated me into the "clean your plate chubby club," while also getting angry that I ate too much, what a dichotomy and confusing contradiction aka mind-funk. I shifted that "mind-funk" into mindfulness. I'd send the hungry kids good energy while reminding myself that a healthy, happy me can help the world from my overflowing cup, but polishing off an extra-large XYZ isn't benefitting anyone.

I had to help myself first; as we first need to put the oxygen mask on ourselves prior to assisting others. I was working with my body instead of against it for the first time in my life. I experimented with what worked and didn't work for me; astonishingly, I was feeling fabulous. I learned that I LOVE INTERMITTENT FASTING! After a few weeks of practice, it became fairly simple, and along with the number on the scale going down, my energy was going way up. My aches and pains were decreasing as my stamina was steadily increasing. Intermittent fasting was the greatest thing since sliced bread. I could even have bread within moderation, too. My eating window was and usually still is in the evening: I'll have a shake or a snack, fit in my workout, then eat a meal. That's what consistently works for me.

With all the time saved by not eating, thinking about or prepping food, I'd have time to live, heal, and learn. I'd "live" by enjoying new experiences or things and playing with my kids. I'd learn about healing, personal development, sexual health and wellness, trauma, psychology, food science, and a lot of "woo-woo" and spiritual stuff, too. Two to three orgasms a week adds 7 to 10 years to a female's life. Um, I want to live forever. I learned about self-pleasure; I had self-punished for enough of my life. Orgasms help release feel good chemicals in your brain, too, which also reduces eating. Intermittent fasting and orgasms were like the weight loss fountain of youth combo, instead of eating Combos.

Exercise also leads to longevity and is a component of the fountain of youth. I started exercising because I love myself. Instead of looking at it as a punishment, it's a reward. What's the best kind of exercise? The kind you will actually do! The at-home workouts were a great start and I enjoy doing them in the privacy of my own home. I worked up to doing bi-yearly resets/detoxes; the clarity and energy astounding-ly demonstrate how when and what we put into our mouths affects us tremendously. A major factor in my improved well-being is having anti-cancer pro-immunity salads, soups, and teas a few times a week. Shopping at my local grocery and health food stores with my detailed list of ingredients is crucial to my success. I wish I had the list early on but, you know what they say, better late than never!

I joined a gym and was mortified at my first attempt on the elliptical machine. I cried because I couldn't even last five minutes, then went through a drive-through with tears streaming down my face. Since my fasting window was around that time, I consciously relished every bite. Astonishingly, I stopped eating when I was full and, shockingly, craved fruit/veggies after a few bites of "junk." Now that's miraculous progress for me at the time! I went back the next day and envisioned adding minutes daily until I progressed up to an entire hour; I conquered my arch nemesis and won my Olympics! I cognizantly enjoy what I eat now. I work out because I care about myself, no longer exercising in a chastising way; however, I had to "work in" versus "work out" to begin.

Nobody becomes 100+++ pounds overweight for "fun." There are virtually always feelings, emotions, sensations, and underlying trauma we haven't processed/healed. I remember crying many times wondering "what the funk is wrong with me"! I had to shift it to "there's nothing funking wrong with me. I did my best post-traumatic experiences, which included horrible coping mechanisms, and as detrimental as they were, they did enable me to endure and cope. I started saying, "Body, thank you for keeping me safe." Instead of disgust, I would look at myself with love and compassion. I created my "I AM" statements/affirmations, including, "I am fit, flourishing and healthy." I learned grounding and self-regulation. I discovered that certain food such as 'bread' and its cousin 'bread' ignited my insatiable hunger and lead to binge-eating. I stopped keeping trigger tempting food at home. I'd have it while out and during my window of eating. Side note: if you live with humans who eat "junk" and you know you'll cave to the crave, Intermittent Fasting is a Godsend when you keep it "safely" within your eating hours. If you don't feel safe, then you'll often self-sabotage, and self-sabotage is self-protection! It's a survival tactic tied to your nervous system.

When I started getting more attention and men flirting with me, I gained back some weight. My nervous system was responding to a past threat. Your nervous system is responsible for keeping you safe, and my survival response to avoid risk and exposure was that I held on to weight. Knowing that, I can regulate myself to get out of the freeze, guilt, fight, flight, shame, eat, spiral. I can "see" what's happening and make different choices. I also choose to delay versus deny. I do not deprive myself of life's pleasures, delayed gratification in lieu of self-deprivation and deprecation. When I delay eating XYZ, I often no longer want it, and will crave a healthier alternative. If I still eat the "junk," I eat remarkably less of it while savoring every scrumptious second of the savory succulence with love!

You're meant to love the skin you're in, and even though I consciously love all of me every day, I wish I didn't have quite sooooo much skin to love. (After losing over 100 pounds, I have a lot of excess skin, so if you're friends with Dr. Nowzarden from *My 600 Pound Life*, or another phenomenal surgeon, please connect us.) I used to feel like such crap. I now use the "crap" as fertilizer and I feel amazing! I look at the skin as a "scar"/winning badge of honor of what I've survived. My story (with battle scarred skin) of how I've overcome what I horrendously went through, can hopefully become a part of someone else's survival guide and a piece to their road map for success and healing.

I've lost well over 100 pounds and became/still becoming "more" of me by "breaking" many of the traditional eating "rules." I'll never "diet" again. I've lost significant amounts of weight and found/created my magnificently authentic self. There's no one size fits all for eating; however, Intermittent Fasting is amazing for most people: It gives your digestive system a chance to rest and your body then has time/energy to heal, resets your mitochondria, reduces inflammation, and if you've struggled with losing weight, it may be your "magic bullet." An orgasm, an apple, exercise, and Intermittent Fasting every day just may keep the doctor away and the pounds at bay.

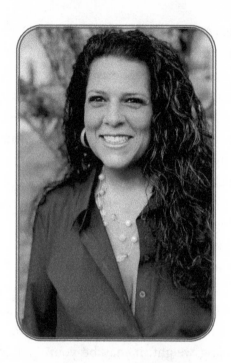

JACKIE FITZWATER

Jackie Fitzwater is affectionately known as the weight-loss whisper-er and the orgasm-whisperer. She is a weight-loss coach and sexual health educator/consultant.

Jackie is a determined woman who knows what she wants and goes after it. After realizing that following someone else's dream was creating her self-inflicted nightmare, she turned down internships to The Nation-al Institute of Health and The White House to focus on her own dreams.

As a grandmother, she returned to school with her adult daugh-ter where she earned a Dual degree and a certificate in Dietetics in the Honors Program at Prince George's Community College, as she represented Native Americans at the United States Department of Education.

As a domestic abuse thriver, she uses her experiences and training as a shaman to help herself and others find freedom. She is intuitive, empathetic, and trauma-informed, making her an incredible healer. Jackie loves sharing her skillsets and tools to help others free themselves from whatever holds them back.

Having lost over 130 pounds, Jackie loves helping people discover their gifts while excavating buried treasures. She currently resides in between Maryland and North Carolina while homeschooling her daughters and practicing "conscious parenting."

If you'd like a copy of Jackie's anti-cancer pro-immunity salads, soups, and teas, connect with her at www.JackieFitz.com.

Chapter 11

FASTING WITH FLEXIBILITY

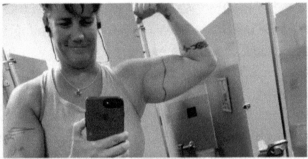
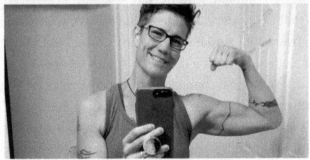

(Top) 2018 - at the gym before IF
(Bottom) 2020 - 2 years into IF without going
to the gym

by Joan Bish

When I first heard about Intermittent Fasting (IF), I distinct-ly recall doing an internal eyeroll. Little did I know, I was about to embark on a journey that would change my life and alter my relationship with food. If you're rolling your eyes, that's okay, but keep reading. You might just connect with one of these stories and it might just change your life.

We live in a world where society has made it incredibly easy to be unhealthy, where "fast food" is fast and usually cheap, but rarely good for you. In our constantly busy lives (where we barely have 30 minutes for a lunch break), we often prioritize eating anything versus eating nothing because we've been taught from a young age that three meals are required to be "healthy." We often don't realize how poor our relationship with food has become. We eat because we're hungry, but we're never really satisfied, so we *keep eating* (hint: remember this thought for later). We become trapped in a cycle that's almost impossible to break free. Almost.

I'm here to tell you that *it is* possible to break the cycle. *It is* possible to lose weight and keep it off. *It is* possible to eat wonderfully satisfying meals, complete with dessert, and still lose weight. But *it is* something that takes work and dedication and understanding. It will not happen overnight. And it will only work when you're an active participant. It's not a wish…it's a decision. And if you're at a point where you've decided to make a change, then this chapter is for you.

In this chapter, I'll explain what worked for me and what didn't. I'll share how I manage fasting with a chronic condition and the epiphanies I have had along the way. One thing I can't recommend enough is having a solid support system. I was successful because my amazing partner, friends, family, and online communities supported me along the journey. **Find a tribe**, they will help you through the darkest times.

~A Little About Me~

I have always been a fairly active person. Give me a warm sunny day outside any time! I love learning something new, going on adventures, traveling, exploring and creating (jewelry, wood art, whatever my brain can dream up). I used to play sports. I used to go the gym *a lot*. At just over 40, I've also seen my share of hard times. I have a genetic abnormality that has plagued me my whole life. I have always been chronically broken. But it wasn't until I was 39 that I learned about Ehlers-Danlos Syndrome (EDS) and Hypermobility Spectrum Disorder (HSD). EDS is a group of genetic disorders that affects the body's connective tissue. For those wondering, the easiest way I've found to explain my situation is that my ligaments are too loose, and my muscles are too tight. My body is constantly at war with itself, and the cost has been steep. I've had more subluxations and dislocations than I can count; 12 surgeries, 10 screws in two body parts and more rounds of various medications than I care to remember. I've done all the treatments and seen all the people. I have all the oils. I've read the books. I've joined the groups. The reality of my situation is that I get to look forward to a future of pain and more surgeries. And I could be really down about that, but I'm not. It's not without its dark days. But I'd rather try to find the light.

~How I Came to IF~

Seems funny now, but I can thank my broken body for putting me on the path I'm on. Seeking relief for my damaged spine, I came across an amazing massage therapist (and fellow rockhound) Mandi Carrasco, who introduced me to IF. With usually 1-2 months between sessions, I started noticing how she was getting smaller and smaller but looked very healthy and vibrant. She told me the secret (IF!) and I rolled my eyes. But I kept seeing her and seeing her progress and the truth is, it's hard to deny that something works when you see the result right in front of you. She pointed me to

Gin Stephens' book *Delay, Don't Deny* which I immediately bought, read, and found comfort in. Gin's concept of **delaying** certain foods, instead of **denying** them, was revolutionary for me. She has since released two additional books (*Fast. Feast. Repeat.* and *Clean(ish)*), which are full of valuable, easy-to-understand information and I highly recommend reading them.

Seeing how successful Mandi was with her fasting and having read Gin's book, I decided I stood nothing to lose from trying (except weight). I was at 198.6 pounds when I truly started my IF journey and was 6 weeks post-op from my second lower back surgery (my 11th overall). But I was determined to do this. It took me several weeks to really get going because I loved creamer with my coffee (more creamer than coffee), and I wanted to transition to black coffee. It took a little bit, but now I can't imagine coffee any other way!

I started with a 16:8 fasting schedule (16 hours of fasting with an 8-hour eating window). I did this because I was used to eating at least three times a day, but truthfully it was more like eating every hour of the day. It was important to me not to shock my system so the very

---

"Am I eating this because it makes me feel good? Or am I eating that because I feel bad?"

---

first thing I did was put structure around my eating habits. This also helped me identify what my eating habits were, which led me to my first epiphany.

Understanding the relationship we have with food is critical; not just recognizing what we eat and when we eat, but *why we eat*. This was a concept that I initially didn't fully understand. One of the most eye-opening realizations I had is that I use food as a coping mechanism for chronic pain. Living in constant chronic pain is terrible. And somewhere along the way I learned to distract myself with food. I didn't even realize I was doing it. But, as I started putting structure around my eating windows, I started to identify these strange cravings that would often hit me out of the blue, which shined a light on the habits I had developed to cope. A spoonful of peanut butter before bed; sitting in bed with chips and salsa. Handfuls of chocolate whenever I felt down. Seeing how I used food led me to my second epiphany. A habit *is a routine of behavior that is repeated regularly and tends to occur subconsciously*. In order to break a bad habit, you have to first recognize and then acknowledge that it's there. Only then can you retrain your brain.

People ask me how I got through the cravings, how I was able to beat that voice in my head telling me to reach for the snacks. As with breaking any bad habit, you have to be in a position where you truly want to break the habit. Your *reason* for wanting to change needs to be stronger than any of the sabotaging thoughts your brain will throw at you. For me, I think about how truly uncomfortable I was in my own skin. And that's enough. You have to find a reason that's stronger than your desire to fail. When I felt the urge to reach for the snacks, I simply recalled the **feeling** I had of how uncomfortable I was. It was a good deterrent for me.

It didn't take long for the pieces to click into place and I was able to move to a smaller eating window (I settled on 23:1 because it works for my life). I approached IF like a big experiment. I paid attention to what and when I ate, how much I ate, and how I felt the next day. Cause and effect. It kept the process interesting. I also weighed myself every day.

While this process worked for me, *it does not work for everyone.* If you obsess over the scale, this might not be a method for you. For me, being able to correlate the numbers on the scale to the food choices I made the day before helped me understand what worked for me and what didn't.

Things that worked:

1. A big salad with lots of veggies, unsalted sunflower seeds and diced avocado;
2. Lean protein (chicken, pork), veggies and jasmine or brown rice; and
3. Avocado ice cream with Lily's chocolate chips and homemade strawberry sauce.

Things that didn't work:

1. Having my window open too long (I tend to overeat);
2. Pasta;
3. Sugar;
4. Alcohol; and
5. Not drinking enough water.

I learned through trial and error that certain things I absolutely love, I can't control myself with (hello spaghetti). In the beginning of my journey, I had to delay these foods (specifically any kind of pasta and all cookies, candy and generally sweet treats) for a longer period of time until I was able to control myself with them. I started eating cleaner; less processed foods and more foods I had to cook from raw foods. This is where it gets tricky.

I said in the beginning that we live in a world where it's easy to be unhealthy and that's absolutely true. For me to give my body the best chance it had to run at its peak, I had to put thought into my meals. I had to cook more, which meant going to the store more frequently for fresh veggies. But my body responded beautifully by melting the fat off and developing lean muscle. It took 8 months for me to lose 65 pounds. I was the healthiest I'd ever been.

But health for me is a slippery slope. On the outside, I usually look healthy and happy, almost glowing. But underneath, my foundation is full of cracks. I'm often held together with duct tape, super glue and a LOT of hope. And sometimes I break. When that happens, I have no choice but to undergo rounds of medication or sometimes surgery. The result of that is an interruption to my fasting. There are several medicines I will never take on an empty stomach. Unfortunately, when I break, it usually means my fasting goes on hold. And you know what? It's okay. Because I can just as easily start fasting again when the medical emergency has passed.

IF is a process. It's the accumulation of consistent practices. It isn't undone in a day or a week, but it can be undone over several weeks or months. IF isn't a diet; it's a lifestyle. One of the best qualities is the flexibility you can have with it. But just like everything else, it takes work, dedication and conscious decisions to be effective.

Thanks to my underlying medical issues, I can no longer go to a gym and work out. But I can take daily walks. I found this to be a key contributor to my weight loss. It's also great for mental health. Getting up, moving, changing the scenery all have positive effects on the body. For me, walking when I was deep into my fast helped me burn even more weight through ketosis.

To summarize, I was successful because I:

1. found an eating window that worked for my life;

2. ate foods that made me feel good and **satisfied** me;

3. drank plenty of water;
4. took walks when I could;
5. found a support system; and
6. experimented and made it fun!

Intermittent fasting is a daily experiment that can have lasting effects if you let it. The only one stopping you from succeeding is yourself. So, get out of your way!

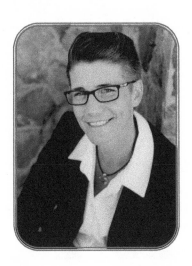

JOAN BISH

Joan Bish is a self-proclaimed jack of all trades and a master of some, currently residing in the mid-west. When she's not working or spending time with her partner and family, Joan enjoys making custom jewelry, Lichtenberg (fractal wood burning) wood art, resin art, honing her lapidary skills on any number of stones she's collected through her past adventures, and traveling when possible.

Joan has been an intermittent faster since 2019 and has enjoyed sharing her story, including the successes as well as the trials and tribulations, with her friends, family, and her online support community. "Intermittent Fasting taught me how to approach things with a different perspective and how to tweak as I go. Not everything works the first time around and sometimes we have to adjust on the fly. The trick is to keep going! Learning this lesson, I've been able to apply the process to different areas of my life allowing me to enjoy success in different ways. Because of Intermittent Fasting, I have certainly Gained by Losing!"

You can check out her musings from inside the bubble "The Unbreakable Will of the Perpetually Broken"
at https://perpetuallybroken.home.blog/.

Chapter 12

FAST LIKE ME

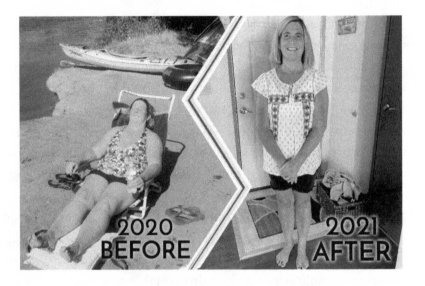

2020 BEFORE — 2021 AFTER

by Julie Stone

I was thin when I was young, but began gaining weight when I was 35, ten years after I had my son.

Additionally, after being diagnosed with depression, I gained weight from my doctor's prescription. It seemed that no matter what I did, including changing what I ate, I always went back to my earlier eating habits. We all have habits; mine was food. What can I say? I love food. I just couldn't seem to get it together.

I tried several different programs including Jenny Craig® and Nutrisystem®, but, at their high costs, I could only afford a month. As soon as I stopped those programs, I gained all the weight back, plus more.

As of the writing of this chapter, I am 5 feet 6 inches tall and am 57 years old. When I began Intermittent Fasting, I was 218 pounds. I knew I would benefit greatly by losing weight, not only for my confidence, but also for health reasons.

After being introduced by my sister to Gin Stephens' books *Delay Don't Deny* and *Fast, Feast, Repeat,* I began to understand why I ate the way I did and that diets simply do not work. I knew I needed to make a lifestyle change and was hoping IF would be the solution. For the first time after gaining all that weight, I learned how to control my portions for my new One Meal A Day (OMAD), snack and dessert lifestyle. I was pleasantly surprised to have discovered that I released 63 pounds and I was feeling much better. My health improvements were immediate.

It was exciting to be on a program that was easy to follow. By adopting an Intermittent Fasting routine, I began to lose the pounds quickly. The weight reduction was a safe two to four pounds per week. Even though some people say you shouldn't weigh every day, I do. I like being accountable and weighing myself daily keeps me accountable to myself. Even with occasional plateaus, I continue an Intermittent Fasting lifestyle and eventually the plateaus level out and I start reducing weight again. Only one year and three months into this routine/habit, I had released 63 pounds.

I continue with my daily IF routine and have a goal weight of 145 pounds. I plan to keep the weight off by adhering to my IF eating routine and walking on the beach four days a week.

The main feature of IF that I like the most is that it works with my boyfriend's eating schedule, whereas before IF, it was hard to get our schedules together and I always felt left out. Additionally, it's much easier for my family and friends to adjust their eating routine to fit my schedule.

What I've gained by releasing all that weight is that I can now breathe easier, I look and feel much better, I can walk on the beach for miles without being out of breath, I wear summertime dresses and don't feel self-conscious about it. Overall, I'm simply a much happier person when I go out in public and, at age 57, I feel more attractive when I'm shopping.

I've lost 63 pounds doing Intermittent Fasting, doing 19:5 OMAD. I feel younger because I look younger and have gone down 5 pant sizes, wear smaller tops, and look good in shorts again.

Previously, I would turn to food when I was under stress. Now, though, I have different outlets when I'm under stress and no longer allow food to pull me under its spell.

I have met a lot of great people in IF support groups online. My doctor acknowledges my results and appreciates my efforts to be healthier. Last year I flew to Puerto Vallarta, Mexico, by myself and met some family members there. I never would have had the confidence to do that when I was heavy. I met a lot of nice people on the airplanes and in the airports.

IF is not a diet; it is a lifestyle. By practicing IF on a daily basis, I have my life back.

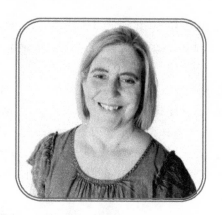

JULIE STONE

Julie Stone is the mother of a wonderful 32-year-old son and has 3 cats that she loves. She enjoys the great outdoors, as well as reading. She realized two years ago that she had to lose weight and keep it off, especially for her health. She needed a lifestyle change that would allow her to live a regular life instead of a sedentary life of pain and depression.

After growing up in Hesperia and Victorville, California, and being employed as a grocery store checker, as well as a caregiver at an assisted living home, Julie married at 23 years of age and had a son. Three years later, after divorcing, she moved to Shingletown, California, with her son. She continued working in Redding, California, and stayed in Shingletown for 11 years.

In 2002, Julie and her son moved to Brookings, Oregon, on the southern coast. Her parents moved to Brookings in 2001 and Julie wanted to be near her family.

Julie is now 57 years old, 5'6" tall and weighs 155 pounds. She started doing IF April 10, 2020, and released 63 pounds in one year and three months. Her goal weight is 145, but her body is happy at 155. The IF and OMAD lifestyle have worked so well for her that it's only natural that she will continue with it forever. She does 19:5 or 20:4 with one meal a day, one snack and one small dessert. She will never go back to her old dieting habits.

Connect with Julie on Instagram here
https://www.instagram.com/jleann65/.

Chapter 13

FASTING FOR MENOPAUSE: HOW I GOT MY SPARKLE BACK

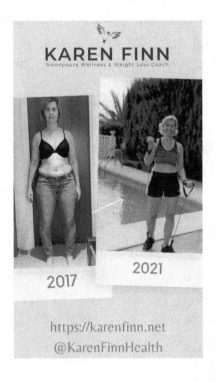

by Karen Finn

The physical and emotional changes that come with menopause can be quite a shock. I know they were for me, especially as it happened early. You may be wondering why I'm writing about The Change in a book about Intermittent Fasting.

Well, my IF (success) story is closely intertwined with my menopause journey.

I started having menopausal symptoms around age 39, the first being sleep problems. At the time, I was juggling a busy career and two toddlers. Naturally, I thought the sleep issues were due to my life circumstances. I'd always thought menopause meant hot flashes and that's about it.

The effect of sleep deprivation – and unbeknownst to me at the time, my declining reproductive hormones – soon began to rear its ugly head. I couldn't concentrate at work, I was constantly feeling irritable, and I had no energy to exercise. My cravings for cakes and cookies were spiraling out of control and working in an office where people were always bringing in sugary treats made the temptation hard to resist.

The weight started piling on, so I decided to try a keto-type diet which focused on cutting out carbs and sugar, eating a lot of protein, and having almost no fruit or vegetables for the first few weeks. Although I lost quite a bit of weight, I felt awful and it wasn't sustainable. Strangely, my breasts started to get very tender and I developed some lumps, so that's when I decided to end the diet. I went for a mammogram, which fortunately was all clear. When I went back to eating normally, my breasts went back to normal, too. How strange is that? This was my first inkling that my diet had an impact on my hormones.

Once I stopped the diet, I gained back all the weight I'd lost, and then some.

Meanwhile, my list of menopausal symptoms continued to grow – crippling fatigue, full-blown insomnia, irritability, brain fog, memory loss, a strong sense of overwhelm and doom, loss of libido, and vertigo, to name a handful.

I tried loads of other "get healthy" regimens, including week-long smoothie and juice detoxes, point-counting programs, and a program that involved very expensive shakes combined with some dirty fasting – they all promised this newfound energy, great health, and weight loss, but nothing really delivered a sustainable solution. And I was miserable when I was doing them. I always felt totally grumpy; I never got that promised energy and never felt any better, even if I lost the weight temporarily.

When I was younger, the weight would stay off, but now the weight was creeping back up as soon as I stopped whatever program I was on at the time. And exercise didn't make much of a difference in terms of weight, whereas before I could quickly get leaner within a couple of weeks of working out more.

I think it's important to mention that although I was above my ideal weight by around 15 pounds, which probably doesn't sound that bad, the real problem was how I *felt*. I felt like I was about 90 years old, and I'd lost my zest for life – my sparkle. I felt frumpy and unsexy, and just wanted to sleep all the time. It was like I was wading through molasses, both physically and mentally.

This went on for a few years and by the time I was 43, I was really struggling. The penny dropped when I started having hot flashes all day long, as well as night sweats that would leave me changing the sheets at 2am. A "good" night was when I slept for two hours in a row.

I finally went to the doctor for a blood test, which confirmed that my hormone levels were "what we would expect to see in a 65-year-old woman." Just like that, I was postmenopausal at 43. The average age for women to reach this stage of their lives is usually around 51, so I felt very alone as none of my friends were going through this yet. My kids were only 5 and 7 years old, yet I felt like their grandma.

Like many women, I didn't know much about perimenopause or menopause besides the classic symptom of hot flashes. Because my birth control had stopped my periods years before, I didn't have the irregular periods that are usually a tell-tale sign that you're in the run-up to menopause.

I therefore had no idea that I'd been going through perimenopause for years without realizing it. Having my second child at 38 also confused things: how could I be losing my fertility when I'd just had a baby?

(By the way, menopause itself is just one date: the one-year anniversary of your last period. After that day, you are postmenopausal. The time leading up to menopause, where your reproductive hormones are on a downward trajectory while fluctuating wildly, is called perimenopause. This can cause all kinds of debilitating physical and mental symptoms and can last for years. For some women like me, symptoms can also continue when they're postmenopausal.)

After the diagnosis, I was left to my own devices and spent several years trying *everything* to feel better and keep the weight off. While I didn't have loads of weight to lose, I couldn't stand the feeling of my clothes getting tighter, and that affected my self-confidence and my mood. My main goal was to *feel* better, both physically and mentally.

Besides all the diets and detoxes, I tried countless supplements and natural remedies, had numerous medical appointments and blood tests that concluded there was nothing wrong with me, hired a natural health guru, and had loads of complementary therapies. Despite all of this, I still didn't feel like myself.

It wasn't until I turned 50 that I stumbled upon the answer: Intermittent Fasting.

I belonged to an online menopause support community and there were always people posting about their hormonal weight gain that wouldn't budge no matter what they tried. One woman mentioned Gin Stephens' first book about IF, *Delay, Don't Deny*, and said it had changed her life. I bought the book on a Friday, read it over the weekend, and became an intermittent faster on that Monday.

It was a big adjustment for my body. I started with a 16:8 fasting protocol (i.e., fasting for 16 hours with an eating window of 8 hours) and it wasn't easy at first, but I stuck with it. Within a couple of weeks, I noticed that my face wasn't as puffy and friends started commenting on my appearance, saying that my skin looked great, and I looked younger.

One friend said that I was de-aging before her eyes and wanted to know what my secret was. Of course, this was very motivating even though I hadn't lost any weight yet! When you start fasting, the body will heal internally before the weight starts coming off. I believe the first thing that the fasting addressed was my inflammation, and "de-puffing" was one of the visible results.

I started seeing some weight loss around the third week, but then I was due to go on vacation. I tried not to worry and resolved to do my best. I managed to fast at least 14 hours and I gained some weight back, but when I got back home, I went back to 16:8 and I got back to my pre-vacation weight within a week. It was so relieving to know that I hadn't completely derailed all my efforts.

I went on to lose a total of about nine pounds within the first two months on 16:8, so I stuck with that until I plateaued after about three months. I did some longer fasts to try and restart the weight loss – the longest one was 36 hours – and that seemed to get things moving in the right direction again.

I then went back to anywhere between 16- to 20-hour fasts and lost about five more pounds, but kept gaining and losing the same few pounds over the next several months.

I wasn't too concerned as I was happy with my weight by then, but I decided to quit sugar for a few months and the weight stabilized. This was about a year into IF, and I decided that I was in maintenance; in other words, I wasn't actively trying to lose any more weight.

Since I've been in maintenance, my weight has continued to fluctuate by a couple of pounds. I usually fast from 16 to 18 hours, but I try to do a 22- to 24-hour fast every so often just to keep my body guessing. I'm not very prescriptive about my fasting and I just try to listen to my body's signals and be kind to myself.

Aside from the weight loss, there have been plenty of what we call non-scale victories or NSVs. The NSVs are what helped me to reach my ultimate goal of *feeling* better.

Once Intermittent Fasting became my lifestyle, everything else started to fall into place. It got so much easier to take control of the other areas of life that have a huge impact on menopausal health: nutrition/gut health, physical activity, sleep, and stress.

Some of the NSVs I've experienced include improved sleep, more energy, more stable mood, intuitively eating the foods that are good for my body, decreased cravings for sugar and processed foods, better blood results (lower cholesterol and triglycerides, A1C levels (diabetes risk), and C-reactive protein (inflammation marker)), no more plantar fasciitis, greater mental clarity, improved vision, and less severe hay fever symptoms.

I also feel like my relationship with food has changed for the better. I no longer have the diet mindset of being "good" or "bad" because I've eaten certain foods. It's so liberating!

By the time I was 50, my friends were also experiencing menopausal symptoms. Knowing that I'd been traveling down that road for quite some time, they started turning to me for advice and guidance. When they saw my physical and mental transformation, they wanted to know more.

It got to the point where most of our conversations were focused on menopause, particularly the stubborn hormonal weight gain that just wouldn't budge. Many of my friends later decided to try Intermittent Fasting under my guidance, and they haven't looked back.

I'm convinced that Intermittent Fasting lays the foundation for a healthier, happier menopause, not least because you'll never have to diet again. It's such an easy way to get your joy for life back, not to mention finally reaching and maintaining your ideal weight. I wish I'd known about it all those years ago.

Now that I've got my sparkle back and feel (and look) younger than I did a decade ago, it's my mission to help as many women as possible to do the same, without spending years searching for the answer like I did. That's why I became a menopause wellness and weight loss coach.

Before I sign off, here are some quick tips about starting your IF lifestyle:

➢ Start with a protocol that's realistic and build up gradually.

➢ Be kind to yourself and if you can't push through, don't give up. Just start again tomorrow.

➢ Just try the fasting part at first. It may be too overwhelming to give up junk food and start fasting all at once. Eventually, your body will intuitively crave healthier options.

➢ Don't compare yourself to others because there will always be someone who's fasting longer and who has lost more weight or has had more amazing NSVs.

➢ Remember that IF is a healthy lifestyle with a side effect of weight loss. It's important to be patient and understand that there may be a lot of healing going on inside your body before you release any weight.

➢ Find and join a supportive community. It can be incredibly helpful when you have questions or need a pep talk.

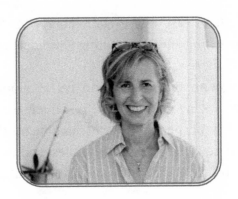

KAREN FINN

Karen Finn is a Menopause Wellness & Weight Loss Coach who is passionate about helping women get their "old selves" back – the ones who felt vibrant, fun, sexy, and had a zest for life. She has been navigating these waters for over a decade after experiencing an early menopause herself. Intermittent fasting transformed her menopause and she is now on a mission to help women tackle their menopausal weight gain and other symptoms like insomnia, brain fog, joint/muscle pain, digestive issues, hot flashes, night sweats, and mood swings.

With Intermittent Fasting as the foundation, Karen supports women to unlock their potential for a happier and healthier perimenopausal/menopausal journey. Karen's clients appreciate her compassionate yet effective approach, which is firmly grounded in the "you-know-yourself-best" philosophy.

If you find yourself looking for a supportive community, join Karen's Fasting4Menopause Facebook® group.

Connect with Karen at https://karenfinn.net.

Chapter 14

FEELING EMPOWERED AS A TRAVELING "IFER"

by Krysten Maracle

Until now, at 58 years old, I thought that I would be on and off various diets for the rest of my life. Luckily, I met Paige Davidson (co-author of this book) at the end of September 2021 at the #1 Networking Event in the World, "Secret Knock." Both Paige and I were signing books at the book signing event for *Invisible No More; Invincible Forever More: Inspiring Stories from Women Who Have Gone From Invisible to Invincible*, in which we both wrote a chapter along with 27 other collaborating authors. After hearing directly from Paige about her 110-pound weight loss journey, I was so impressed that I asked her if we could stay in contact after the event and work together. Little did I know that less than six months later I would be writing a chapter about Intermittent Fasting (IF) in March 2022 after being coached by "Coach Paige."

You may be thinking, "How can Krysten Maracle even think she can be an author with authority or claim to be an expert on the subject of IF in less than 6 months?" This is a great question! The same question I had for Coach Paige before I accepted this privilege to write this chapter. Coach Paige said to me: "Don't you remember how ecstatic you were when you returned from France at the end of December after being gone for almost an entire Month (December 1 – 23, 2021) stating that you ate and drank your way thru France (Nice, Cannes, Monaco, Lyon, and Paris) and did not gain ANY weight.

This was a "Maracle." Let me explain.

My previous trips to Paris in December, my birthday month, were always strategically planned! I learned that one month before my departure date to "regimentally" succumb to the Atkins' diet in order to lose 15 to 20 pounds. I did this since I had proven over all the previous 8 or 9 visits to Europe in December that I would gain 15 to 20 pounds while on vacation. Yes, you heard me correctly! I would pre-lose weight before my trips since I routinely gained all the pounds back while traveling abroad.

In addition to this trip to France in 2021, I also went on a cruise to Mexico for a week (October 16 – 22, 2021) and traveled to Sedona, Arizona, for a week (November 14 – 21, 2021). Thankfully, I returned from both these vacations with the same outcome: No weight gain after 2 weeks of travel! Believe me, this I felt was another "Maracle." Just to clarify, I ate plenty of food as well as enjoyed my cocktails and wine on both occasions while in Sedona and Mexico. During the cruise, I definitely indulged with the 3 course meals at dinner plus desserts along with 1 or 2 glasses of wine. I did not diet either on land or at sea. All I did was regulate my eating timeframe, not what I ate or drank. I really did put IF thru the "ringer" and the "test"!

For the record, I am not a doctor. Like all advertisements, please consult with your healthcare provider on your specific needs. None of this content presented in my chapter is doctor's advice. My experiences shared in this chapter do not guarantee the same results for you. This information is merely for you to think about and decide for yourself if these ideas and/or techniques could support you in any fashion.

My main emphasis for this chapter is to illustrate my goals of IF and the reasons why I never need to diet again. My goal for IF is two-fold. First, while I am living at home in La Jolla, California, I will be using IF to lose weight gradually, nothing drastic. Two months after submitting my chapter, on May 21st, 2022, I have the pleasure of hosting a wedding shower for my daughter Kaitlyn and her fiancé Brody in my backyard. On September 4th, 2022, I will be the "Mother of the Bride" as we celebrate at 4 Points Farm in Sevierville, Tennessee. Luckily, these two lifetime events are a huge incentive to encourage me to work IF with variety, so it is not monotonous. Secondly, while I am on travel, my IF goal is NOT to lose any weight but rather to maintain my weight. Luckily, a no weight gain to me is a success since vacation is a time to indulge in the pleasures while not over-indulging.

I am so thrilled that dieting for me is gone forever because I have proven to myself repeatedly that IF works. This is not to say if you enjoy your specific diet that your diet is wrong. Again, this is merely my observation in just the last few months since I discovered Intermittent Fasting (IF) with Coach Paige. I have learned that the diets I previously followed were never the "solution" for me since diets eventually come to an end. Diets are simply temporary and not long-lasting. For me, any diet worked until I could not maintain all the "rules" of what I was allowed to eat and what I was forbidden to eat. Simply stated, "A diet for me was not sustainable over time." Furthermore, many diets that I tried were confusing since they contradicted other diets. So which diet is correct? Which one is best for me? How do I know?

For example:

- Atkins™: Eat fatty foods. Eat meat, eggs, cheese, butter, etc.
- Vegetarian/Vegan: Do not eat fatty foods. Eat nuts, fruits, vegetables, etc.

It would take me too much time to compare all the diets out there (Keto™, Mediterranean, Dukan™, Ornish™, Dash™, Flexitarian™, etc.) but, unfortunately, all these diets have a list of "Good" and "Bad" food while on their specific diet.

Luckily with IF, I do not have to categorize food as "Good" or "Bad" ever.

I am free to choose my food as I desire each and every day. IF is mainly about the time "window" that you eat and less focused on what you eat. Of course, I am not claiming that you can eat fast food every day with 3 desserts during your eating window and expect to lose weight. Common sense must still be applied! Most people know what is nutritional and what is not.

IF is the first eating lifestyle, not a diet, in which I am empowered to be my own boss both while eating at home and traveling abroad. I am in FULL control of what I eat. There is no "sin" food. I simply choose when and how often I eat depending on my end-goal; I only need to be concerned about my eating window's duration. Will my eating window be long or short today? The great news is that there is no WRONG or RIGHT answer. How awesome is that?

With IF, I have so many different eating "windows" (timeframes) options that fit my lifestyle depending on my activities and social calendar. I find that "18/6" (i.e.,18 hours fasting and 6 hours timeframe to eat) is the easiest for me. However, some days I have a shorter eating window (20/4) while other days have a longer window (16/8).

Each day is a NEW "IF" routine if I choose. Notice how I chose the word "routine" instead of diet. This is a lifestyle change, a new routine, and I get to choose my routine on a daily basis. I decide if I want to create the same or different eating window as yesterday, or the day before yesterday, or not. This flexibility makes IF so refreshing and versatile. As a result, I know I can perform IF for a lifetime and know that I will be SUCCESSFUL.

Once I know my eating window, I decide what I want to eat. I found that keeping a journal (either on my phone or on paper) encourages me to make better, healthier food choices. This documentary process gives me awareness in which I can discover patterns that work for me, or not. My feelings and mindset can also be jotted down as well to keep data on my mood, energy level, and mental clarity.

With today's technologies, many IF apps are available on your phone for either free, monthly, or a yearly charge. I use one called Zero and love it. It's easier than carrying around a journal. I personally like to physically touch a button to "start" my fast as well as "stop" my fast. It somehow makes it feel "official," sort of like a starting line and finishing line at a track meet.

Other tools that I have found to be helpful are books/audibles, podcasts, and social media groups. I love audio books and have both *FAST. FEAST. REPEAT.* and *Delay, Don't Deny* by Gin Stephens on Audible.

As a worldwide traveler by visiting over 24 countries Costa Rica, China, Canada, Turkey Mexico, Ireland, Italy, Australia, Austria, Germany, Belgium, Greece, France, UK, Netherlands, Croatia, Bulgaria, India, Malaysia, Singapore, UAE, Bahamas, Hungary, Czech Republic (and many countries multiple times), I want to give you hope that you can maintain your weight not by WHAT you eat, but WHEN you eat. I want to emphasize that even if meals are not made at home and eating out is a regular occurrence (due to working or vacationing), there is Intermittent Fasting. You are still the boss of what you eat and the beverages that you drink. No diet needs to be a dictatorship in your life.

Every day I make choices and am in control of those choices. I have been choosing more water and even have a new mantra, "I love water"! I choose to eat slower and stop eating BEFORE I am totally full (especially at Thanksgiving). I find that I can stop eating when I am about 80-85% full. If needed, I give myself a 30-minute "lapse period." If I am still hungry after 30 minutes, I may eat more until I am satisfied completely. This really makes me feel great. I never DENY myself food anymore like I was forced to do while on various diets.

For the first time in my adult life, I am empowered with food and feel so much more freedom. I enjoy the abundance in this life and enjoy making daily choices about my eating window. Should it be a shorter or longer eating window? Again, I DECIDE!

I hope and pray that by sharing my experiences it has given you hope and inspiration to change from a diet to a new IF lifestyle. I have gained so much wisdom through this short time of Intermittent Fasting and I want you, if you desire, to discover it for yourself!

Thank you "Coach Paige" for all of your support and patience with me. Much appreciated.

Stay Safe, Stay Healthy, and Stay Blessed. Namaste!

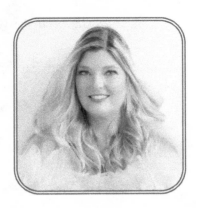

KRYSTEN MARACLE

Krysten Maracle was born in Point Loma of San Diego, California, and graduated from San Diego State University with a Computer Science degree with Honors in 1987.

She worked as a navy civilian at "Navy Information Warfare Center Pacific" in Point Loma for over 30 years, retiring from the Cyber Security Department in 2019.

Due to Krysten's upbringing as an Incest "thriver," she has a passion to help women achieve their goals regardless of their traumatic past and wants all women to know that they are WORTHY just for being born.

Because Krysten has lost so many close people to suicide (her only sibling, brother Bryce, her maid of honor and other close friends), Krysten wants to share HOPE to all people, young and old. Everyone matters and deserves to thrive and find happiness. Krysten has discovered that forgiveness is key.

There is always a new day, EVERY DAY. Never give up!

Today, Krysten is a mother, speaker, and Bestselling Author of the following books: *Power of Proximity, Wealth Made Easy, Momentum:*

13 Lessons from Action Takers Who Changed the World, and Invisible No More; Invincible Forever More.

Please feel free to contact Krysten on Facebook® messenger at https://www.facebook.com/krysten.maracle.

Chapter 15

THE FREEDOM AND FIERCENESS TO FAST FOREVER

by Lisa Fischer

George Michael belted out "Freedom" in 1990, and the song has given me ear worm ever since. Of course, this isn't a time for an existential discussion of that song, just of the catchy tune and lyrics that flood my head space.

It's my nod to Intermittent Fasting, actually. It is, in a word, freedom. Freedom from the constraints of diet dogma. Freedom from meal planning. Freedom from the condemnation of the scale. No more counting calories. No more counting steps. No more checking in with others on what I had eaten that day or week. No confessions. No shame. Just freedom.

My journey begins 20 years ago when all of the sudden, out of nowhere, my thyroid went kaput. I gained maybe 10-15 pounds after a quick loss of weight (sometimes the gland is overactive before its ultimate demise) so I was up about 10 pounds from what was comfortable. Then another 10. I was diagnosed with several autoimmune conditions around the same time (vitiligo, anybody? It's often in the same autoimmune family with Hashimoto's thyroiditis). But I couldn't figure out the weight thing. I did the diets; my favorite was the HCG diet where I took human **chorionic gonadotropin drops twice** a day combined with a 500-calorie diet. It was the unicorn diet, for sure. But after the diet, those 18 pounds that fell off in three weeks came charging back like a mad grizzly bear, and I was as hungry as one, to boot. That's what caloric deprivation does. It just makes the rest of the body mad. Our Creator didn't want us to fret at what we should wear or eat (Matthew 6:25), nor that we might eat too many or too few calories. We do best when we eat in an ancestral way so that we never have to check the back of a package or enter into an app how much we've eaten. Eat in a time-restricted manner and watch those concerns dissipate.

Back to the freedom part. In 2017, my college son had come home for Thanksgiving break and was telling me about the podcasts he would listen to on the seven-hour drive from Louisiana State University in Baton Rouge, Louisiana, (Geaux Tigers) to Little Rock, Arkansas, our home. He asked if I had heard about Intermittent Fasting and the Intermittent Fasting Podcast, to which I replied, "If you are telling me this because you think your mother needs to lose weight, you won't see your 23rd birthday" (he was 22 at the time). He said, "No, Mom. I'm telling you because you like things that deal with health." What could be HEALTHY about starving yourself? I pondered. He told me a very skeletal format for fasting (don't eat again until 12:30pm tomorrow and it was 6:30pm when he and I had the conversation). And I ripped off the Band-Aid and did what he said. The first 72 hours were weird almost. By day three, I was really hungry, but I did not die. I had been instructed by well-meaning medical professionals and personal trainers to eat five small meals a day. I was told to drink stevia-flavored water in the morning (I'm not a coffee drinker and had hot tea with cream and sugar many days). I nursed those drinks all morning when I was an on-air morning radio personality for the state's top contemporary hit radio station. Then when I left the station, I would eat nuts at 9:00am, lunch at noon, snacks at 3:00pm and dinner at 6:00pm. AND I WAS STARVING. If you asked me how I was, I often answered, "Hungry." From what I know now about insulin's effect on my hunger hormones, I know why I was always hungry. Insulin stokes, not the embers of metabolism like we were told, it rather stores fat and makes us hungrier. Of course, it is a life-giving hormone, and I don't want to diminish its importance. But I want you to see that too much of it gives us many of the modern diseases we hear about today.

So what about living a life that reduces the release of the all-important insulin hormone to maybe 4-6 hours a day? What's that about? That's about longevity, cancer prevention and treatment for type 2 diabetes, actually. (My attorney wanted me to tell you that this isn't medical advice). But what it is instead is my advice on how to feel great and never fret about your weight again. As you know, this is Intermittent Fasting.

Back to freedom. My friends who are chasing their calories burned on their wrists via their Apple Watch don't feel free. In fact, they are in bondage because they can't stop their workouts until they hit a certain number of calories. The people who count their calories all day and look at the back of bags for nutritional advice, they, too, are tethered to numbers and not living. I am living with Intermittent Fasting.

I lost about 10 pounds in about five weeks with fasting. I had a 6-hour window of eating what I wanted in that time allotment. I now mix things up with longer fasting windows followed by shorter ones. Our bodies love it when we do that! I am post-menopausal and a thyroid patient as mentioned earlier, so my metabolism is far from impressive. But my body has adjusted to this season of life, and I weigh what I did about 30 years ago when I started having children. The magic of body recomposition is impressive. Though my weight isn't what I'd love for it to be, my size is smaller than it has been in years. I'm 5'8" and weigh about 150 lbs. I was 143 lbs. when I married in 1988, but who cares what the scale says? I am just telling you because when I read these testimonies, all I want to know is, BUT WHAT DO YOU WEIGH? We over identify with that number on the scale. What we should be measuring is our vitamin d, fasting insulin (huge connection to longevity-people in the health space like that at 5 or 6, mine is 2.2), blood pressure and how much sunshine and sleep we get. Those are the real indicators of good health, not that dumb number on that dumb scale.

I remember when my bestie saw me a month after I began this journey, she asked, "How long are you going to do this thing you're doing?" I replied, "Forever!" She blurted out, "Lisa Fischer!" It was like I was in trouble. She said, "You're always doing all the diets. Isn't this just another one?" I knew in December 2017 that it was a forever thing for me. I said, "I will never go back to all-day eating. Why would I when I feel so good?" That's what fasting does-it provides energy, mental clarity, better skin, less anxiety, less hunger, quicker satiety and better sleep. Remind me why I would want to return to being sluggish, sleepy, always hungry with worse sleep?

My autoimmune conditions have improved immensely but aren't cured. My rare swallowing and motility disorder is the best my advanced clinician gastroenterologist has ever seen (it's called achalasia and is very rare). He was the one who pointed out, "We were never designed, as humans, to digest all day. By giving your esophagus a break, you have definitely improved a potentially serious condition."

Food used to dictate my life; now it is there for fuel. Delicious, life-giving fuel, without worry of calories or macros. I live a life free from the worry of where my next meal will be or when I have to eat it. I love this life and love the freedom it has given me. Want the freedom that fasting gives? Start today.

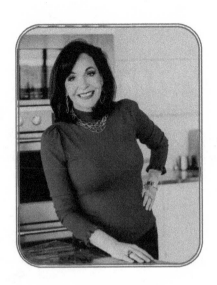

LISA FISCHER

L isa Fischer is a longtime radio/tv broadcaster and journalist from Little Rock, Arkansas. Having spent more than half of her life in front of a camera or microphone, she believes she is the face of Intermittent Fasting in Little Rock. She's a magazine editor, podcaster, website author and health coach who helps people overcome weight gain, hormonal imbalances and fatigue. She and her husband Kris have been married since 1988 and have three adult children and two really cute granddaughters.

Reach out for more information at
https://lisafischersaid.com/intermittent-fasting/.

Chapter 16

FROM FOOD FEAR TO FOOD FREEDOM

by Lisa Glick

My name is Lisa Glick. As I write this, I have just turned 62 years of age! I was born in March 1960.

Right now, I'm a petite, fit, active woman. I run, hike, dance, sing, and lead a very active positive life.

This was not always the case.

As a young child I was always moving. Skipping, dancing, playing, ice skating, water skiing, swimming, singing, gymnastics, and many other things. I was always fit and muscular. I ate when I was hungry, stopped when I was full. I looked adorable in clothes. I felt great about my body. I felt great about life.

About age 9, I remember starting to have mood swings for no reason. Some days I'd feel joyful and other days I'd have a dark feeling of doom hanging over me. As I got older, the mood fluctuations were mild and manageable, but the darker days were getting darker. I was very musical and theatrical and thought it was just part of having a creative nature.

As I got into my teens and stopped growing, I started putting on a bit of weight. The summer after 9th grade I started jogging and "cutting calories." I lost about 15 pounds and I looked and felt great. Going back to sophomore year in the fall as a cheerleader I received many compliments on the weight loss. This was the mid '70s when thin was in and thinner was even better. I kept restricting, over exercising and, like many others, I was heading down the path of anorexia and disordered eating. I remember enjoying the restricting, and feeling that was the one thing I could control in my life. This went on for a while until one day my dad forced me to step on the scale. My parents started monitoring my food and I sort of got it together. In the '70s, there was no counseling or therapy for this "thing."

I went away to my dream college for Music Education as a voice major. The depressive episodes increased. I went to college at age 18 at 110 pounds and left four years later at 160 pounds!! Somewhere during my sophomore year, I started adding in some of the sugary treats I had avoided for years, and I couldn't stop!! I felt possessed. The weight gain was awful and made me even more depressed. I had no idea at the time that the depression was causing the binging. I graduated college, started my job as a public school music teacher, and somehow managed to stop the binging. I went back to running, cut out snacking, and counted calories again. I was actually doing some Intermittent Fasting at the time without realizing it. I'd delay my eating until about 3:00 in the afternoon and felt fabulous.

I met my first husband in 1984. We courted and married in 1986. In 1989 we welcomed our daughter. I thought I had the most wonderful life. Fabulous pregnancy and delivery. I was madly in love with my baby and my life. I was home on maternity leave and loving every minute. As the months went on, I started to experience anxiety and depression. Once again, I had trouble eating and sleeping. I got thinner and more anxious as the months went on. When my daughter was about a year old, I had a nervous collapse. I had a day where I just could not function anymore.

I was hospitalized for several months with no improvements. I was like a guinea pig for different meds. A year plus of different doctors, different meds, different treatments, different diagnosis, and no change. Finally, I found a woman psychiatrist that correctly diagnosed me as Bi–Polar and put me on Lithium. SHE SAVED MY LIFE. Two weeks after I started the Lithium I was almost back to my old self. It was quite remarkable. I could feel the medication clearing up my brain. After almost 2 years of incorrect diagnoses, this was a huge gift.

I slowly started building my life back. I went back to work, taking care of my child, enjoying my marriage, and contributing to society again. As I became better, I started adding in some positive health tools. I was running, performing, doing community service, and cleaning up my food. I started cutting out sugar and carbs and eating more whole foods. I was not just living; I was thriving.

For about 18 years, the Lithium served me well, but there were side effects. Since I was managing my life so well, my doctor helped slowly wean me off the Lithium. I added in more good fats and protein. I spent more time outdoors. I worked on managing my stress and anxiety with therapy.

My first marriage slowly ended in 2013 and I survived that grief. During the divorce once again I had trouble eating and sleeping, but kept it in check. After the marriage ended, I went through my menopause and gained some weight mainly in my mid-section. I felt scared that I was going to blow up again. At this time, I was starting to run Ultra Marathons (50 kilometers) and I needed to improve my nutrition. This was when I was introduced to the Ketogenic lifestyle–using fats as fuel.

At first, like many women, I was petrified to add the fat back into my diet. I decided to trust the process. My hormones were very messed up and my cortisol was high from the stress of being single again and navigating a new life after 28 years of marriage.

Keto was a game changer for me on multiple levels. It immediately reduced my anxiety. My belly fat started to improve. My running improved. I found I could go longer distances without constantly eating. My entire outlook on life improved.

Once I became fat adapted, fasting occurred organically. Fasting and Keto combined made me feel like wonder woman. I loved the freedom of IF and not worrying about food all day. I loved eating to satiety and never leaving the table hungry. IF truly gave me appetite correction. I was able to get back in touch with my hunger and satiety signals. Fasting also gave me even more mental clarity than just Keto alone. As a singer, fasting helps with my creative process and keeps my voice healthy from the autophagy.

AUTOPHAGY. This is the absolute best thing about fasting. As an athlete, fasting has helped with my recovery. As a post-menopausal woman, fasting has helped with hormone regulation, skin elasticity, libido, and general well-being. Fasting helps me get in touch with my feelings and manage them in the moment. Since I'm not focusing on food all day, fasting frees me up to live my life to the fullest.

My fasting schedule varies depending on my activity level. I can do multiple hours of hiking or running fasted. I can perform and teach dance fasted. I have a very flexible schedule. Most days I average 16-18 hours of fasting. Some days I go 20-24 hours. Occasionally, maybe once a week I break my fast mid-morning after about 14 hours. Once a month or so I may do an extended fast.

Now at age 62, I have transitioned from Keto to full on Carnivore in combination with daily IF. I've been Carnivore for a year and 3 months as of the writing of this chapter. I was having some issues with bloating and digestion, so I decided to try carnivore as an elimination protocol. I felt so much better eliminating the vegetables with oxalates, lectins and other anti-nutrients. What? The girl that lived on huge bowls of veggies and salad has changed to a meat-based diet! I now feel like I am on the best food plan for my physical and mental health.

As a long-distance runner, I often get push back from other runners about fasting. I will never go back to eating all day long. Fasting has given me peace. Fasting has given me freedom from food anxiety. Fasting has helped this 62-year-old body stay active and fit. Fasting gives me clarity of thought. Fasting gives me spiritual gratitude for the little things. Fasting has greatly improved so many aspects of my life.

Humans were not made to eat every few hours (or minutes). The cavemen went days sometimes without food while hunting. Calories-in versus calories-out is an antique concept. Good health is about reducing insulin. Fasting keeps our insulin low which helps prevent many diseases.

I am incredibly grateful that I have been able to recover from disordered eating through Intermittent Fasting. I hope my story can help you.

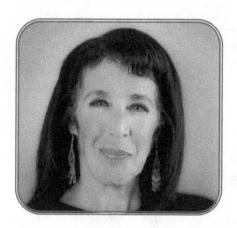

LISA GLICK

Lisa Glick is a retired vocal music educator. She is an avid hiker, trail runner, and dance fitness teacher. Lisa is a vocalist and performs at many local venues in Arizona. Lisa is originally from New York but now lives in sunny Arizona.

You can connect with Lisa Zucker Glick on Facebook® or Glicklisa on Instagram®.

Chapter 17

NEVER GIVE UP ON YOURSELF!

by Lou Jensen

I am a member of several Intermittent Fasting support groups on Facebook®. You could say that I had immersed myself in these groups for quite a while, taking it all in. I saw testimonials of success like I had never seen before. I was fascinated, but still I only observed. I saw quite a few group members lose over 100 pounds. Over time, I saw jubilant pregnancy announcements from women who had been suffering from Polycystic ovary syndrome (aka PCOS) and had started doing Intermittent Fasting specifically to balance their bodies' hormones and be able to conceive. They joyously shared that they would see all of us again in nine months. I saw several people reverse fatty liver disease, a multitude of people whose health markers improved to their doctors' amazement, and yet I continued to observe and not take the leap. Finally, someone from one of the groups specifically invited me to begin my Intermittent Fasting lifestyle – that very day.

She encouraged me to just give it a try. She said Intermittent Fasting offered an ideal way to lose weight, that I could begin today, there was nothing to purchase, no special foods that I had to eat, I could use the foods that I already had in the house, and it was free! Furthermore, there was no counting calories, or macros, or points, or anything else, and there was no food prepping, and no weighing or measuring foods. As I read all of these benefits of Intermittent Fasting, I realized there really was no downside. I strongly believed in myself and knew that if I decided to do it – I could certainly do it! I had seen all the amazing health benefits (although I am extremely healthy and had always been). Before my recent cataract surgery, I had not been to visit a doctor in over 60 years. No need to, because I am never sick, not even so much as a cold. But I did want to lose a few pounds and that was my motivator. My only hesitation was that at first I did not believe that Intermittent Fasting wasn't a diet. Over the years, back to the age of 19, I have always been obsessed with wanting to lose a few pounds. I never had a massive amount of weight to lose, but I was always trying to lose those few pounds in order keep my weight from getting totally out of control. I firmly believe that had I not dieted all those years, at this point I would be as big as the side of a house! I tried diet after diet after diet and am of the firm belief that whenever anyone chooses to lose weight, once that way of eating was eliminated (and all diets are eventually eliminated), whatever was lost is regained, plus more.

After sitting on the fence for over a year, I decided to take the leap. At the age of 83 and standing 5 feet 2 inches tall, I hold my weight well. I was never 'fluffy,' but have always been solid. I looked pretty darn good! But I have always, all these years, strived to lose that 20 or so pounds that I carried around and wasn't comfortable with. That 20 edged up to 25, which became 30, which led to needing to lose 40+ pounds. I started Intermittent Fasting May 12, 2020, wearing a tight size 16 pants. I wasn't intimidated. On the contrary, I was totally on fire. You see, I had something many people didn't have. I am a strong, confident woman with great self-esteem and great determination. I didn't hope I could lose the weight; I knew I was going to lose the weight.

I started out like gang busters. Before I started Intermittent Fasting, I noticed that many people started really seeing big results around the three-month mark. This led me to decide to look at the big picture, and not worry so much about how much I lost each week, if I had a small loss, or even the occasional gain. They do happen sometimes, and they can be very hard. Each day I would plan and write out my food for the next day, and each day I followed that plan without any alterations or add-ons. This kept me from grabbing foods randomly and it has been a wonderful strategy for me. I did so well that I lost 40 pounds in five months. I couldn't be more thrilled and was about 25 pounds away from the goal weight that I had set for myself. And then it happened.

The mother of all plateaus! Of course, I knew about plateaus and I even expected them to happen. I was not concerned for quite a while. But as this plateau stretched on for months on end, I kept losing and regaining the same 5 pounds. Eventually I kept losing and regaining the same 6 pounds, then the same 12 pounds. I tried tweaks in my foods. I tried varying my fasting times. I even tried extended fasting, where you fast for longer periods of time than your usual daily fasts. My longest fast to date has been 27 hours. At no time, however, during this long period of time, did I lose faith in myself, nor was I tempted to quit. I decided that maybe the missing piece of the puzzle was an accountability partner. I have seen lots of people hook up with an accountability partner and it is often very helpful to both partners. I tried a few partners, but they all fizzled out after a period of time. I felt dissatisfied because I felt like I was doing all the cheering for my partners, but not receiving any cheering in return.

It was at this point in my journey that I was approached by one of the co-authors of this book to share my story. I was confounded. Who, me? While I had done well there for a while, I had been mired in this very long plateau. What in the world did I have to contribute to this book? I hadn't lost a huge amount of weight like others had. To save my life, I couldn't think of a single non-scale victory that I could identify. However, after considering it, I had a change of heart. Here I was, starting Intermittent Fasting at the age of 83 with complete confidence that I would succeed, while many in their 50s and 60s felt defeated at the thought of starting their fasting lifestyle, because they thought it was too late. I had done well, which proved that I could do it. I didn't have that much left to lose, and I knew how to make tweaks. One thing is for sure; success is nothing more than a few good habits, practiced consistently. Every day. I have the discipline, determination, and grit to continue to consistently practice my Intermittent Fasting lifestyle and reach my goal. Consistency is the one thing that can overcome any obstacle. From day one I believed I could do it, and I continue to believe I can! I never stopped trying and I am so glad I found Intermittent Fasting. So, I decided to say YES to writing this chapter.

I said yes because I can't say enough good things about Intermittent Fasting. I would shout it from the rooftops if I could. It is the easiest way to lose weight no matter what your age. I was 83, so I am proof of that, and it doesn't matter how much you need to lose. It works for everyone if we put in the work. Mostly, if one word I say in this chapter inspires even one person to begin Intermittent Fasting, lose weight and get healthy, it would absolutely mean the world to me.

Once I did say yes, the very first thing I did was to say "Jesus, take the wheel!!" The next thing I did was to consider my daily habits that are healthy and continue them with consistency. I use visualization and imagine myself at a smaller size. Just a little smaller, not anything unrealistic. I drink water daily. I have a pretty floral water bottle that holds 22 ounces that keeps my water ice cold and the bottle doesn't sweat. Plus, using the bathroom all day makes me feel "thinner," so it's all good. I continue to plan my food for the next day and follow that plan faithfully, with no deviations. I have a book of affirmations that I have been adding to for years. If I ever have a down day, I read my book until I find an affirmation that resonates with me on that day. This is so helpful for my mindset and attitude. I continue to follow the adage, "Compare yourself to yourself to measure progress.

Compare yourself to others for possibilities." I also walk, between 6,000 to 9,000 steps a day.

Some tweaks that I have made lately are helping, apparently, because last month I lost six pounds! I decided to alter my eating window to be earlier in the day. I am practicing an 18- to 20-hour fast and am enjoying closing my window by 4:00 or 4:30 pm. I love not eating late. For breakfast I have been loving having eggs with veggies plus a yogurt, then later have veggies with protein and a protein shake. While I don't count calories, I am aware of them and have been having around 1,100 calories or so each day. This is keeping me satisfied. I was adding fruit to my smoothies and yogurt, but decided to cut that out. I also was grabbing a small handful of pretzels during my window but have chosen to cut that out as well. And the last tweak that I have made I am thrilled with. I found an accountability partner and we just seem to click. We are both very encouraging of each other and cheer each other on. We both made a list of what we want to do and accomplish, and our lists are very similar! We both have similar amounts of weight to lose, and this partnership has fired me up and I am energized and so excited to work together with my accountability partner as we both reach our goals. I highly encourage you to find a great accountability partner, as well as to BE a great accountability partner. It makes the journey more fun and productive.

I will close by saying that I am now 85 and wear a very comfortable size 10. I have recently had cataract surgery in both eyes and my vision is amazing. I have lost a few more pounds, which is thrilling. These updates, especially the size 10 pants, make me happy and keep me going. I WILL get there. And what if my body is already at its happy place? I am comfortable and happy with where I am; I will continue Intermittent Fasting for the rest of my life, and if down the road I eventually do make it to goal, fantastic! If I stay right where I am, I am healthy, happy, and blessed.

Oh, and that surgery I had on my eyes. In preparation for it I had to get a physical for the first time in 60 years. Imagine my elation when I discovered that all my health markers are in healthy range (ok, so I am a little bit low on vitamin D – an easy fix☺). I am on a mission, to continue to practice Intermittent Fasting, to remain healthy and energetic, and to be a role model to other women, both my age, older, and younger.

Together we are well. Together we win!

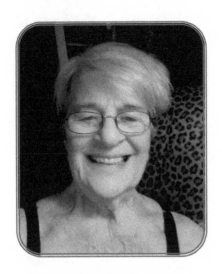

LOU JENSEN

L ou Jensen, at age 85, lives a serene life. She has two children, five grandchildren, and seven great grandchildren. She was self-taught in painting folk art and primitive designs. She dabbled in home improvement for the past 50 years and created a faux brick wall by using joint compound, paint, and the tool used for taping sheetrock seams. It is one of the unique things she takes pride in accomplishing single-handed, at age 79. It measured 20 feet long by 9 feet high. Lou spent 30 years being self-employed, creating old world crafts such as dolls and Santas that she sold at shows. The materials used to make her crafts were all either given to her or purchased at antique shops. She presently paints artwork on recycled furniture, giving it new life, and maintains three huge flower beds that she created several years ago.

Chapter 18

A NEW SONG IN MY HEART!

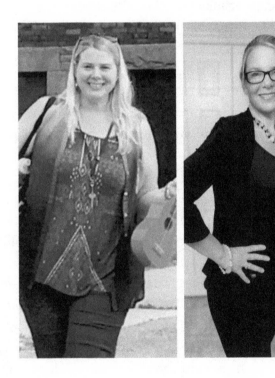

by Monique Coretti

H i, my name is Monique. I'm from Ontario, Canada. I am grateful for this opportunity to share my newfound hope and restoration from a lifetime of chronic struggle with dieting and weight problems. In short, I went from trying almost everything, giving up, and then finding the miracle of Intermittent Fasting (IF) which has given me a new song of life. A new tune that's given me a new rhythm in my step, beat in my heart, dynamic for living, theory on wellness, and rest in my soul.

I grew up in Montréal, Québec, Canada with my mom and older sister Michèle. When I was about eight years old, our uncle asked my mother if her daughters were overweight because she starved herself to give us extra food. That joke launched the start of my confusion and struggle with body image and my awareness of being obese. Getting in on the joke, I also blamed my mom for giving us fudge to eat every time we felt upset or cried, but sadly it was true. Food was comfort. Our mom stayed single and struggled with her own addictions as an alcoholic and workaholic, which meant we were home alone most of the time where food became our close friend and favourite pastime. Our father, who lived in Ontario at the time, would come for seasonal visits centred around elegant restaurant dining which led to conversations about our life goals, appearances, body shape, and the importance of looking good. What he thought of me started to matter more and more the longer I went without feeling his unconditional love.

Even though I felt lonely and rejected at times, I found contentment and joy in the creative arts. I was blessed to have great extra curricular activities and hobbies to keep me occupied. I took part in many art programs and immersed myself in singing lessons at an early age because I loved to sing. At age 13, our family doctor handed me a food tracker and calorie value chart and told me to eat no more than 1,000 calories a day to help me lose weight. It worked. Yet, I still did not understand healthy eating. It did not seem to matter that I was only eating a cup of ice cream worth 350 calories each night for dinner. What seemed to matter most was the scale going down. This was often celebrated with extra attention and praise from my parents and family. My diet issues led me to experiment with diet shakes, puddings, lentil and cabbage soup diets, and non-fat food plans. At sixteen, I started singing professionally at a dinner theatre, performing lead parts in front of thousands of people, and travelling with the Montréal Symphony Orchestra Chorus. I had an agent who gave me many great opportunities to work towards a stage career; however, he told me that although I had a pretty face, I would need to have a body that matched. At auditions, I was asked how easy it was for me to lose weight, which led to perpetual yo-yo dieting and paltry programs. I would get the part, diet myself into costumes, finish shows, then party hard until I was back where I started. I eventually moved away to study Musical Theatre and, in desperation to maintain my weight there, joined many weight loss clinics and even had a boyfriend help me plan out calorie-restricted diet plans. I was 'white knuckling' my way to maintain a normal weight for years. In my third year of university, I tore my ACL and was on crutches for several months, returning home at an unhealthy weight of 200 pounds. My weight issues led me to pursue a new interest in performance. I had been training with several world-class opera coaches and decided I might as well pursue that route instead of trying to be the Musical Theatre 'triple threat' that can sing, act, and dance that I was not quite cut out to be.

I moved back in with my mom to attend McGill University in Montréal. I started a new round of Weight Watchers®, got a gym membership, and reached my 'life membership' goal by the end of that year. By now, something shifted in me. I started to look for greater meaning in my endeavors and I pondered on what my impact was in the universe. I was now displeased with the competitive side of my newfound career and its pressures, such as trying to be a size six. What I was looking for was a deeper purpose for my life. I decided to return to praying to the God of the universe I had grown up believing in, rather than to the universe itself, and ask Him for direction. These prayers were answered immediately when my friend Tellie moved into my apartment building and called me from the hospital. Her vision was impaired after emergency eye surgery. I gladly helped her out with some daily tasks, running errands, and was very open to read to her Bible devotions when she requested my help. I was inspired by her great faith and the trust she had in her loving heavenly Father and knew God was present as we prayed and read His word together. The strongest message I learnt was from Isaiah 41:10. I was not to fear or be dismayed, for God would strengthen me, help me, and uphold me with His righteous right hand.

The word of God comforted me more than any other teaching I had heard of, read, or studied. I feared life, making decisions, and being the one in full control of my own destiny. I started to experience and understand God's infinite love for me, His healing power, His amazing grace, mercy, promises, and truths. I now had an absolute to anchor to, a purpose. I no longer had to concern myself with trying to 'affirm' my way to success or compete with others to get to the top. I would now simply pray, trust, and love all the people God sent my way, and to those people I shared this radical gift of redemption, sanctification, and transformation. I was now living for eternity, leaving this world's pressures, expectations, and stresses behind, and witnessing God's grace and miracles every day.

My mom passed away three weeks after I married my husband Frank, a wonderful Christian man. Together we have raised two beautiful boys, have written and recorded music that has glorified God, and have led worship for hundreds of church services together. I am privileged to have worked with adults and children to celebrate their unique artistic gifts as a full-time elementary arts teacher and private vocal coach. I also love serving the Lord in women's ministry, kid's church, and worship leading. Since becoming a Christian, I have attended many beautiful services, retreats, and conferences that helped fill my heart with God's destined direction and vision for my life. I worked on being obedient and saying yes to everything He has for me, believing God for healing in every area of my life.

I would love to tell you that my journey has been perfect, full of joy, hope, and peace. But for every mountain-top moment I've had, I've also had to fight out of a dark valley; the darkest of valleys being my continued battle with food. My heart would ache as I struggled with failed dieting and constant weight gain. I had always struggled to surrender my desire for perfection. My vain thoughts of what people thought of me held me in bondage. I would end up losing the weight, but I never lost the idolization of my own body; I viewed myself as a compulsive overeater, as someone who could never find healing. I spent nearly a decade as a sponsor in a 12-step recovery overeating program. I was at my goal weight and was maintaining, but I still suffered from the strongholds of pride, guilt, shame, fear, and desperation. All those years of struggle wore me down. I just wanted to be free from what I can only describe as a vicious, persistent, dark cloud of mental confusion and oppression. I could not diet anymore! I had decided I had enough with this oppressive program and quit. What soon followed was gaining all my weight back and then some. Despite this defeat, I knew that I was headed in the right direction if I kept God as the focus of my life, not the scale. I felt God prompt me to seek first the kingdom and His righteousness. (Matthew 6:33.) I needed to stop and reflect, waiting on God to do a mighty work. I focused on Him alone and surrendered my goals, desires, disappointments, and destiny into His hands. I believed, cried out, and pursued the God of miracles to liberate me. He would, and He could, set me free.

God's miracle came in March 2020. That miracle was Intermittent Fasting.

As a Christian, I was used to reading of the benefits of spiritual fasting but was blind to the idea of it being a lifestyle. I had prayed and fasted one day a week for a season, and occasionally did longer fasts, but it was only in the last few years that I heard about fasting as a lifestyle for wellness. My sister's naturopathic doctor recommended it, so I told my sister I would join her and give it a try. I had nothing to lose. My curiosity led me to study the benefits of fasting and I soon learned about its extreme healing benefits like autophagy (the body's natural regeneration of cells). My previous conditioning to eating six to eight times a day was being challenged by all the science about fasting. Science was teaching me that my metabolism and hormones were compromised by a history of yo-yo dieting, which made me insulin and leptin resistant. (*The Obesity Code*, Dr. Jason Fung.) I immersed myself in the study of time-restricted eating and began fasting sixteen hours a day. Through prayer, the Lord strengthened me to do longer fasts. I found the peace of mind I was longing for. It was the first time in my entire life that I was free from the confusion surrounding food, appetite, self-control, hunger, and weight management. There was now a time to eat, a time to abstain, a time to feast, a time to focus, and I discovered balance for the first time. I found freedom, rest, and healing from my strongholds. I would dedicate each fasting time to God and noticed that I was being healed physically, mentally, and spiritually. During my fasts, I felt a renewed joy a new intimacy with God. I was now hungering for the true bread of life. (John 6:25-40.) My energy dramatically increased, my sleep improved, my chronic sickness disappeared, my mind felt clearer. This was God's answer to my prayers.

My newfound zeal for life led me to connect with other intermittent fasters online. I read several more books including Bert Herring's *AC: The Power of Appetite Correction* and listened to healing stories that all encouraged me to keep fasting.

I am now singing a new song filled with deep joy, contentment, and healing in my heart. I currently try and use a variety of fasting protocols. I have shed lots of weight. I love fasting and am still learning much, fine-tuning, and enjoying the healing process and progress for my mind, body, and soul.

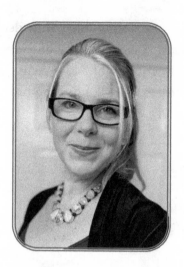

MONIQUE (FOLLOWS) CORETTI

Monique (Follows) Coretti is a Canadian educator, singer-song-writer, recording artist, vocal coach, the bride of one, mom of two, friend of God, and intermittent faster.

Monique explains how Intermittent Fasting has brought her singing a new song in her heart. After over 35 years of yo-yo dieting, she prayed for a miracle and found a new lifestyle that brought tremendous joy, contentment, and healing for her mind, body, and soul. This newfound freedom and her passion for ministry led her to connect with like-minded Christian women. She was prompted to share her testimony to help others still looking for their miracle by commencing her certification as a Christian Life Coach with Leadership Coaching Canada and forming the My Daily Bread of L(IF)e Christian Women's Intermittent Fasting Support Facebook® group. Her prayer is to continue prospering on her fasting journey, share God's incredible ways of healing and restoration with others, and honour the Lord in all ways possible with as much vitality, wellness, and health for His glory.

You can contact Monique at mcbellavoce@gmail.com or find her and her HuzzBand at https://corettimusic.com.

Chapter 19

WHAT IS DIFFERENT ABOUT THIS TIME?

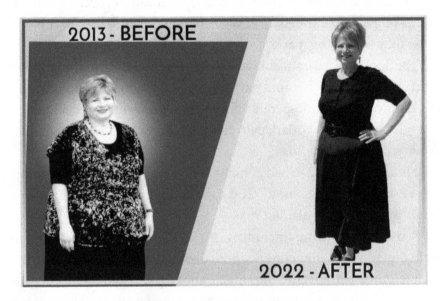

2013 - BEFORE

2022 - AFTER

by Sheree Moon Missionary

One thing I ponder, "What made this time different?" Why has my life changed so powerfully, so that I have a deep peace that obesity is soon to be a thing of my history, no longer my present, nor my future?

Recently I retired from living overseas for 37 years. I loved my life and the work God gave me amongst Filipino children and those who ministered to them. I love the special family God gave me as a single missionary, to raise and love as my own. But my health was declining.

I had lived a lifetime with obesity, constantly trying ways to overcome and consistently failing.

I am 67 years old and 5 foot 1 inches tall and (at least) 308 pounds at my highest, with a long history of obesity. The narrative is that Mom was away for a week when I was six, and Dad fed my brother and me hotdogs. After that I got fat! My poor Daddy—it wasn't his fault, but that is the story. Whatever the root cause—genetics, culture or addiction, I was obese, a food addict. That doesn't mean a broccoli addict! It means pizza, chips, sweets…. If vegetables and fruit were a part of my plate, they were a tiny part.

The food disorders of binge eating, emotional eating, nighttime eating, and bulimia became part of my life. No matter the counseling, diets or my own desperate efforts, these powerful and debilitating struggles were mine. A dark path to walk for any, and for me as a missionary, deeply shameful.

I remember going to bed at night and praying, "Lord, in the morning, let me wake up skinny." God can do anything, but a miracle or magic pill wasn't His plan for me.

I tried everything including prescribed amphetamines as a young teen, weird diet clinics where dreaded sessions worked to associate foods with disgusting smells, shots, packaged diet food programs, and group meetings where the public weigh-ins shamed me further. And then, what felt like the last, desperate straw, a $10,000 weight loss surgery. I lost some, but I learned how to gain it back, because I didn't have healing with my emotional eating or change to sustainable, healthy eating. I learned good lessons along the journey, but so longed for deliverance. That is a strong word, but that was exactly the need!

Sicknesses came in the form of hypertension, arthritis, multiple digestive complications, GERD, painful hemorrhoids, fatigue and nausea after meals. All of these symptoms required more and more medication. This included years of depression and anxiety disorder, requiring more medication.

I became so feeble that the last few times I traveled the long international distances, I had to be in a wheelchair because the twenty-six hours of transit and three airports were so difficult.

Flying became a phobia. Not good for one whose work required frequent flights with up to 16 hours airtime. The real pain caused bruises and included the emotional distress of squashing my seatmates.

The shame, self-hatred, long clinical depression, anxiety disorders, and struggles with hopelessness went as deep as frequent suicidal thoughts. I got to rock bottom.

I want to give God glory for sustaining me all of those decades, living in a hot, tropical country where it is not easy even if you are physically fit.

During most of my service in the Philippines, it was unusual to see an obese person. There are more struggles with obesity now because of worldwide lifestyle changes, but for many years I was quite unique in morbid obesity. Because of cultural differences in speaking candidly about physical issues, folks would often casually comment to me about my size. This was difficult for me, because of my cultural sensitivity.

Hope began to come about three years ago as I learned about nutritional answers that were not "diets" but focused on healthy eating. After researching the side effects of the 15 medicines I was on for my physical ailments (lifestyle choice sicknesses) and the medications for the mental health concerns, I started longing to be off of these medicines. They served me well for many decades, but I felt for me the side effects were now outweighing the benefits. I wanted to pursue lifestyle changes that would bring health.

After consultation with my Christian psychiatrist and primary care doctor, we outlined a plan over six months to wean my body and mind off the prescribed drugs. My need for the hypertension drugs was related to my weight, so I first needed to continue with lifestyle changes to bring my numbers into a healthy range.

I learned about *True North Health Center* in Santa Rosa, California, with Dr. Alan Goldhamer. It is a medically supervised water fasting center, with focus on education in Whole Foods Plant Based nutrition. In August 2018 I began treatment for 13 days. 3 days of preparation of eating their delicious whole foods plant-based menus, then 7 days medically supervised water fast, and 3 days of refeeding. My primary reason for treatment was for healing my brain from medicines, but I had wonderful physical results as well. Autophagy (the benefits of the body healing itself while fasting) was at work.

Valuable training while there reinforced the nutritional changes to reduce my dependency on processed and fast foods.

Weight started coming off, slowly but surely. I learned to enjoy vegetables and fruits. I was breaking habits of turning to chips, fast foods, and sweets that were addictive to me and difficult for me to eat in balance. 'Progress not perfection,' was a big life lesson for me as a recovering perfectionist. Previously, a slip would set me on a spiral lasting days or months. By learning to form habits that worked for me, I was changing, learning grace. The secret for overcoming was consistency.

The struggle was still strong with emotional eating and night eating. I wanted to be free. I REALLY WANTED TO BE FREE. I know Jesus came to give us abundant life with freedom from bondage, and, not just for others, it was for me, too.

I found podcasts, articles (probably algorithms, but glad for these), Gin Stephens and Intermittent Fasting kept popping up. Through her Facebook® groups, podcasts and books, the learning curve began, and I haven't looked back! I started my self-designed "doctorate" in health, reading all I could get my hands on: Gin Stephen's *Delay, Don't Deny: Living an Intermittent Fasting Lifestyle*, and *Fast. Feast. Repeat.* along with Dr. Jason Fung's *The Obesity Code*. In addition, I studied Paige

Davidson's *Fast with Paige,* and Graeme Currie's *The Fasting Highway,* and Netta Gorman's *Life after Sugar* podcast to name a few.

Reading the stories, having support, and receiving affirmation of my own progress on the Facebook® pages was an important part of my journey.

On May 27, 2020, I started Intermittent Fasting. Now, it seems strange how fearful I was. How could I not eat for hours at a time? Baby steps–I decided to stop eating at 10 PM and not start again until morning. 10 hours–that was hard! I was conditioned to eat through the night out of habit, for comfort, and to get back to sleep.

I was 231 pounds when I added Intermittent Fasting to my weight loss journey, having begun by reducing processed foods and focusing on "Whole Foods Plant Based." Since IF, I average 25 pounds lost per year. It is beautiful to see stories of those who lost quickly, but for me, it needed to be different. It has been important for me to go slower. I had much to learn, deep changes to make and healing to experience.

The bondage to my food addiction was intense. During many periods of my life, at any meal, I was thinking of what I could eat next. I went for long periods, always full. I did not know how to experience hunger. Only during sleep would my stomach have a rest, and that often was interrupted when I woke with insomnia and would eat.

Now I was hungry for answers and finding hope. Resources are now abundant and include books, YouTube® testimonials of lasting victory, medical doctors embracing change in treatment for obesity, scientific research supporting Intermittent Fasting plus the benefits of clean eating. I learned of the often unhealthy cultural changes since the '70s, the availability of frozen dinners, fast foods, highly palatable processed foods, and the move toward eating on the run and away from homecooked meals using real food.

Community came through the Intermittent Fasting groups, including the Christian group, My Daily Bread of L(IF)E - Christian

Women's Intermittent Fasting. As more family and friends find IF a great tool in their own health journey, we support each other.

My usual fasting routine is 18 hours with a six-hour window for eating. Longer fasts are sporadically used for autophagy healing.

Intermittent Fasting is a safe boundary for me. After my last meal, I enjoy my ritual of starting my fast on my fasting app. When I press the app, I think, "Thank you, Lord, I have gotten good nutrition today. All my needs are met. There is no need for me to be hungry later, and if I am hungry, it is emotional hunger."

NSVs (Non-Scale Victories)

Very grateful for the pounds lost, but the "Non-Scale Victories" (NSVs) are wonderful!

- Constantly improving emotional health
- Happy in clothes
- Comfortable in booths
- Increased energy
- Lack of pain
- Health and peace about aging
- Enjoy exercise
- (more) Peace around food—still working on that because I am not sure if I can moderate or need to abstain from trigger foods.

My forever plan is to practice the disciplines I have learned. The yummy foods that work for me are plant based, but I have added eggs and fish, while focusing on whole foods, and working to avoid processed foods, flour and sugar especially. Intermittent Fasting is my daily practice. It feels too good. No going back.

I practice my exercise disciplines. I do the vibration plate three times a day with floor exercises and weights. I walk my little fat puppy.

Over the next few months, the focus is to get the additional pounds off. Whether it is 40 pounds or wherever my SLIM body wants to settle.

I am now at 181.2 pounds, having lost a total of 127 pounds. I want the excess fat off my body, to be whole and strong. I will continue to focus on eating real food, not processed food.

The process of reaching my health goals has been slow, but I have come to embrace the steadiness of my weight loss while God makes great changes in my mindset. He could have done the healing overnight, I know, but the changes are deep and needed.

Many of the learned principles cross over in other areas of my life. For example, applying formation of new habits (*Atomic Habits* by James Clear) and overcoming perfectionist thinking.

WHAT HAS MADE THE DIFFERENCE THIS TIME

What has made the difference this time for me? After spending thousands of dollars, desperately determined, but always failing. What is the secret?

- Mindset Change—vigilantly tending my attitude
- Daily practices—Habits (exercise, nutrition, fasting)
- Safe boundaries of Intermittent Fasting—Healing from emotional and night eating
- Keeping "My Why" foremost
- Consistency—returning quickly to baseline, getting back on the horse immediately
- Sustainable, satisfying, yummy nutrition, not feeling deprived
- Focus, with an undivided mind
- Stay alert when tempted for highly processed foods and cultural triggers
- FB— group, podcasts
- Books

- Friends
- Devotions : YouVersion Bible on health & weight loss
- Honesty with myself
- Replacing "reward eating" with other happy activities
- Growing level of Trust and Reliance on God

I know if I can do it, with God's help, anyone can!

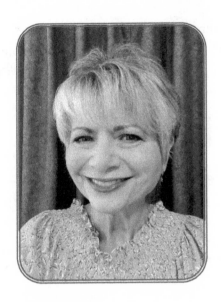

Sheree Moon is a Texan through and through, but with a Filipino heart after serving 37 years in the Philippines as a missionary. She has a wonderful, God-given family of children she was privileged to raise who continue their studies and work in the Philippines.

A graduate from Southwestern Assemblies of God University with her Master of Science, she has been part of a gifted team who developed ministries to children and continues to serve as a long-distance mentor in her retirement.

During her time of service, Sheree helped develop children's discipleship curriculum and programs and served on the board of children's homes, feeding programs, as well as helping to develop training for children's workers throughout the Asia Pacific.

She continues to travel overseas in short-term service as well as speaking in the United States. She loves caring for her puppies, reading, and being an active part of her family's lives in Texas.

A personal priority for Sheree has been learning about and applying healthy living lifestyle changes the last three years. She is passionate about living an overcoming life in her own physical, spiritual, and mental health and being supportive of friends and family on the journey to health, through mentoring, writing and speaking.

Please connect with Sheree here:

sheree.health.freedom@gmail.com

Chapter 20

THE GAINS WAY OUTWEIGH THE LOSSES

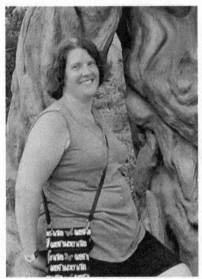 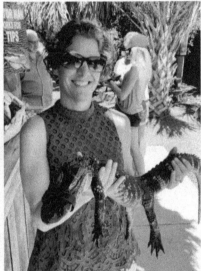

July 2019 - Before IF   April 2021 - After IF

by Sue Schulte

I came to Intermittent Fasting (IF) because of my weight, but gained so much more than I lost. Here's my story...

I went on my first diet at 22 years old. Was I overweight? Not according to my BMI at the time. But I felt fat. I'm 5 foot 7 inches tall and weighed 150 pounds at the time. I cut my calories to 1,500 per day and worked out one to two times every day. I made it to my goal weight of 135 pounds, but it was excessive, and I couldn't keep it up. My weight slowly crept up over the years as I changed jobs, moved states, and got married. By the time I became pregnant with my first son, I was up to 175 pounds. I gained over 50 pounds with that pregnancy, and no doctor ever told me—"Hey, you need to slow down. You're gaining too much weight." Realistically, I knew. But in my head, I blamed the doctors for not telling me. I weighed in at 235 pounds when I had my son. I went back to calorie restriction to try to lose that. No exercise this time. I told myself I didn't have time with a newborn. I made it down to 200 before I got pregnant with my daughter. This time, the doctors told me I wasn't gaining enough. I actually lost a couple pounds initially because I was so nauseous; however, I was back up to 230 pounds when my daughter was born. Soon after, I was pregnant with my youngest.

After three kids in 3 1/2 years, I was ready to get my weight under control. Weight Watchers® was going to be my solution. I lost about 75 pounds on Weight Watchers®, but when it came time to set my final goal, I wanted to set it at 150 (3 pounds below their recommendation). The Weight Watchers® staff told me I'd never get there. I think I used that as an excuse to give up, along with my frustration with being "rewarded" for losing weight by being allowed less food. My brain was struggling with constantly having less and less food. I was always hungry, and the weight wasn't coming off very fast anymore. Anyway, I gave up and worked my way back up to 230 pounds. Over the years since, I've done a lot of calorie restriction, went back to Weight Watchers® a few times, and even took up running a couple times. (My husband is a runner and encouraged that. I ran a few half marathons over the years, but I never enjoyed it, and I never stuck with it.) My weight bounced around between 175 to 230 pounds. I was always either actively gaining weight or actively losing weight. I could never figure out how to maintain.

Enter IF... I first heard of IF in 2018 from a friend at work. I have to be honest, I thought she was crazy. I could never do that. I'd starve...

In July 2019, I was at the end of my rope. I was back up to almost 230 pounds, well into the obese category. I had thyroid problems, asthma, allergies, plantar fasciitis, and my liver numbers were up (AST & ALT) on my labs. I think I had non-alcoholic fatty liver, but the doctor never actually said that. I had no self-confidence. I felt miserable in my skin and avoided pictures at all costs. I hated that I had so few pictures of me with the family but, even more, I hated how I looked in the pictures. That was when I remembered my friend talking about IF. I decided, I can limit my eating to 8 hours a day. I did that for one week – I saw my friend that week and she recommended I read *Delay, Don't Deny* by Gin Stephens. I ordered the book, then went on vacation for a week. I didn't fast on vacation, but when I returned on August 1, 2019, the book was waiting for me, and I started IF that day.

I read *Delay, Don't Deny* and was amazed at all the information. I ordered some of the books Gin Stephens recommended and began my journey into learning about weight, health, etc. At the time, *The Obesity Code* by Dr. Jason Fung made the biggest impact on me. It was the first time I had heard that weight gain was NOT my fault. It was NOT my personal failings that were making me miserable. This was a whole new mindset that gave me the power I needed to embark on this journey. I started IF with a 16:8 pattern (fast for 16 hours, eat during an 8-hour eating window). I quickly moved to 20:4, because I discovered I wasn't really hungry after 16 hours. I settled into an eating window from 4pm – 7pm on workdays and 3pm – 7pm on weekends. I generally ate one BIG meal along with a snack. I've always been a perfectionist, so I set rules for myself. Every day I would fast for a minimum of 20 hours. My eating window would never be more than 4 hours. Once I got past the first couple weeks, it was the easiest thing ever! Every diet I had ever been on consumed my thoughts. I thought about food ALL day: What should I eat? How much can I eat? Can I have more? Is it time to eat yet? With IF, for the first time, I wasn't thinking about food all the time. I also stopped taking responsibility for every meal everyone in my family ate. My kids were teenagers, and able to take care of themselves, so I began only planning and cooking one meal each day and allowing them to take care of their other meals. That removed a lot of stress from my life! It was such freedom! Since I wasn't constantly thinking about food, I now had all this time to think about other things...

I followed that 20:4 pattern for the first year. I saw results pretty quickly, which doesn't happen for everyone. But it certainly kept me motivated. I lost almost 20 pounds in the first 2 months, and over 70 pounds in the first year! I went from a size 18/20 down to 4/6. All my health conditions improved significantly! I went on to lose about 10 more pounds, then actually <u>maintained</u> my weight within a 5-pound range without any effort! I usually kept to the same 20:4 schedule, although I was more flexible with moving my eating window and averaging my fasts. I often did a shorter fast Friday into Saturday, ate lunch on the weekends (instead of dinner), then did a longer fast Sunday into Monday when I switched back to a dinner window. I tried some 36- to 42-hour fasts, and just experimented some. I returned to running off and on, but kept a regular walking schedule. I developed a lot more confidence and started feeling good in my skin.

I'm not perfect, though and I had several struggles along the way. I didn't have much of a local IF support group to help me learn and adapt, so I did a lot of reading and connecting with people on Facebook®. I heard from MANY people that I was starving myself. My family questioned my choices initially as well. However, as people saw my success and improved health, they became far more supportive. In the beginning, I also struggled with visiting friends and family, because I thought people would judge me for not eating with everyone.

What I learned with time is that it was my lack of self-confidence that was causing my problems. No one cared if I ate with them. I was finally able to just enjoy visiting. One of my biggest struggles was breaking the "habit hunger." I wasn't really hungry. But I initially found myself thinking I was hungry at certain times, or when I went certain places. Over time, I was able to break those habits, and rarely struggle with hunger these days. I also gained about 5 to 10 pounds back during a period of high stress in the fall of 2021. In the past, this kind of stress would have led to a much larger weight gain. But this time I had the confidence I needed to make some changes in my life. I found a new job, which I'm truly enjoying, and adjusting to life with far less stress. There are also days when I eat too much junk food (I still have a sweet tooth). I only do it in my eating window. I generally eat far healthier than before IF. I always plan out my one main meal. I've never particularly enjoyed cooking, but it's so much less overwhelming to plan and cook one meal every day, than it was to plan and cook 3 meals every day.

IF has given me so many blessings that I never imagined when I started. I have gained so much more than I lost, and I know I'll never go back! Below is a list of some of my personal gains, which have been life-changing for me:

- Not only am I at a healthy weight... but I've been able to maintain it with little effort!
- I have more energy than I have in years!
- I like pictures!
- My liver is healthy again.
- I no longer need medication for allergies or asthma.
- I need less medication for my thyroid.
- I have found an inner calm... I truly believe that IF is the reason that stress no longer affects me as much as it used to. I find

myself able to approach almost any situation and remain calm and relaxed.

- Optimism – I can find the bright side to anything these days. It used to be so much more difficult.

- Confidence – I truly believe that I can do anything I set my mind to.

- Mindset – really a lot of these gains could be categorized as mindset, but I thought they all deserved their own emphasis. I really think about a lot of things differently than I used to, and I think it all stems from first changing my paradigm around weight.

- Awesome friends! I have met so many people through IF that I never would have otherwise. Through Gin Stephens' Facebook® groups, I got connected with a local fasting group – Measure Me Life – and have met some fantastic people.

- Social life – with increased confidence and self-esteem, I now socialize more than I used to. I have been able to surround myself with a lot of wonderful people.

- Exercise – I always said I needed to find an exercise I enjoy. I have joined a line dancing group! Great people, and so much fun!

Today, I still generally follow a 20:4 schedule. With my new job, I'm up at 3:30am, so I don't eat at typical times. I eat my big meal around 2pm – 3pm. I usually cook dinner for my family in the evening, and if I'm still hungry, I may have a snack while I'm cooking. I don't eat dinner with the family because it's too close to bedtime for me. I keep them company during their dinner and enjoy catching up with them. I'm still maintaining a 70-pound weight loss and currently wear size 4/6 clothing. My current struggle is developing a pattern for regular exercise with my new schedule. I dance two days a week, but am still working on how to best fit in walking and other exercises. I've also continued learning more about my personal health and what foods work best for me. I recently participated in the Zoe program (www.joinzoe. com) and learned about my personal blood sugar responses, blood fat clearance, and gut microbiome. I'm currently attempting to integrate their personalized food recommendations to learn what foods make me feel the best. I'm so excited about how far I've come. But I'm just as excited about everything else I have yet to learn!

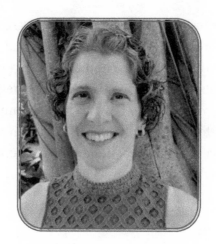

SUE SCHULTE

Sue Schulte grew up in the suburbs of Chicago and now lives near Louisville, Kentucky. She earned her BA in Social Work from the University of Toledo in 1995 and her MSW (Master of Social Work) from Indiana University in 2001. Most of Sue's career has been in the corrections field; however, she is now working in a substance abuse setting. Sue loves counseling and helping people! She has been married for 23 years and has 3 children ~ 2 in college and her youngest is graduating high school in 2022. She never imagined herself as an author, but what a wonderful opportunity!

Sue's hope is that this book inspires others to find the motivation to embark on a journey that can lead them to health, happiness, energy, and optimism.

Chapter 21

MEASURE ME LIFE...
SO MUCH MORE THAN WEIGHT!!!

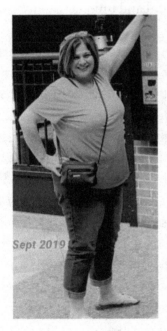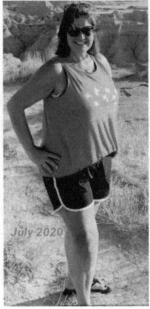

Sept 2019 — July 2020

by Tammy Roach

H ave you ever felt broken? Just felt like you couldn't get yourself together, lose the weight, keep the weight off, fix the problem? I feel
that way often and I'm not ashamed to share my feelings, ask for help,
or pray for wisdom and grace. I don't think we are meant to struggle

alone either. I find great strength in my praise, worship, and fellowship not only at church, but also in my small groups. During a recent sermon at my little church, Southeast Christian in Louisville, Kentucky, I learned about "kintsugi," which is the Japanese art of gluing broken pieces of pottery back together and then tracing the visible cracks with gold. This 400-year-old term was built on the idea of embracing flaws and imperfections to create an even stronger and more beautiful piece of art. When my pastor, Kyle Idleman, used this term as a metaphor for spiritual healing, I learned that in the process of repairing brokenness, God creates something more beautiful and unique than we could have ever imagined.

Of all the non-scale victories I've gained from my Intermittent Fasting journey, the most impactful one has been my spiritual awakening. What do I mean? Well, I think that the experiences I have had in the past two years, since finding IF, have helped me to see myself through my Heavenly Father's eyes. My weight has always been a burden to me, from childhood to post-menopausal-hood. I've allowed this burden to define me for most of my 51 years. Although I'm sure those who love me have never thought a thing about whether I was a size 8 or a size 22 – I can't help feeling broken by the size of my jeans! Through this new lifestyle and many sermons, I have discovered that the one thing I've allowed to define me may just be the one thing the Lord wants me to use as my testimony for His love, patience, and grace. Most every sermon I hear will speak to me about my weight issues, regardless of the topic, and how I should use this struggle as a blessing to help others!

The story of my Intermittent Fasting journey began in November of 2019. After only about four weeks of living this lifestyle, I decided to share how easy it had been for me to lose inches and gain confidence. You see, in the past I had lost and gained weight so many times; almost always gaining back more than I had lost. After trying Weight Watchers® unsuccessfully many, I mean many, times; attempting to keep my weight off after gastric bypass; and the other annual attempts without being able to keep the weight off, I felt like a failure and very broken. I would have never dreamed of sharing my experiences on social media because I felt like everyone knew I was always on another fad diet. But this time was different. I couldn't believe the side-by-side before and after 4 weeks picture. I had finally found what would work for me and it was not a diet but a new way of life. Or so I thought…

Deciding to share my success on Facebook® was the beginning of something bigger than I could have ever imagined. After my post, I had friends who were private messaging, calling, texting, and posting asking me, "How do you do this fasting thing?" My friend, Tammy Scrogham, and I decided instead of replying to each person, we would start a Facebook® group. As the number of members grew rapidly, we decided to host monthly meetings and a Facebook® Live each week to help our members feel engaged and a sense of community. We wanted to share what had worked for us and kept saying if it only helped ONE PERSON to feel better, we had done our job, sharing our stories of fasting and our love of Jesus.

We held our first monthly meeting on Sunday, December 29, 2019, in Hillview, Kentucky, with over 20 friends in attendance. I prayed with the group before sharing my story of finding Intermittent Fasting and my success so far. Instead of using a scale for measuring physical success, we used a tape measure to track measurements and photos to see the differences from month to month. We were on a mission to share a story.

Then the Covid-19 pandemic hit us March 2020. The monthly meetings were halted due to social distancing, but I kept having weekly Facebook® Live meetings within our growing group to help our fasting friends. I also created several YouTube® videos to share my passion. Each week on the Lives I would discuss topics about fasting, how to use a fasting tracker app, how important exercise is for both mental and physical health, while sharing my faith. We even started a chair yoga class that members could attend over Zoom. It was important to keep our community together, especially as we entered an unprecedented time in the history of our world. Even during a pandemic, I felt it was easier to use a clock to clean fast 16-18 hours daily than it was to count calories, steps, carbs, and all those other things we count to lose weight. I can't imagine how much weight I would have gained if not for my new lifestyle. During this year, I was able to lose 45 pounds in 9 months, hitting 199 (onederland) the day after my 50th birthday. On that milestone birthday, I was interviewed by my friend and best-selling author, Gin Stephens, on her Intermittent Fasting Stories podcast, episode 118! As we supported our group, we would say things like "there is no wagon to fall off" or "you fast every day," but we soon learned this may be true, but not for everyone.

In the fall of 2020, Stacy Williams started co-hosting the Facebook® Live meetings and we called it the "Tabby & Abby Show." Stacy and I have been best of friends since we were 13 years old. We had reconnected several times over the years, only to drift apart again. We always picked up right where we left off; that's the great thing about best friends! Having the opportunity to see each other weekly and spend this time together was something we were both passionate about and we felt like we were making a difference to those who were watching our show. We discussed on Lives not only our weight loss struggles, triumphs, and how Intermittent Fasting worked for each of us, but also our private lives and how we could hold each other accountable to live faithfully. It wasn't long until I started noticing something different about Stacy. She was reading Bible based books on self-care, clean eating, and praying without ceasing. She started sharing with our group the notes and lessons she was learning, and we pivoted from an Intermittent Fasting support group to more of a Christian support group. The members loved learning more about our Lord and how HE can make all the difference in our lives. We weren't sure where the Lord was taking us on this journey, but we knew it was something big, something huge to reach thousands of people. As we told our members, "Trust the process," we were not only trusting the process for healing within our bodies through fasting but also our spiritual lives.

Then in 2021, I felt led to create a small business, Measure Me Life, LLC, to help financially fund our meetings, website, and promotional items. However, the business plan was not really a business plan, but more like a nonprofit organization. We were in the business of helping people. We had always given free Intermittent Fasting support and our meetings were free, so we didn't want to start charging our members. We created individualized fasting support and speaking engagements which are offered through the website for a fee, but no one has taken us up on those options. We envisioned our fasting family at churches and community centers all around the country sharing each of our journeys, because we all have our own unique story, all equally important and impactful. Knowing if we could get people to understand and practice the Biblical principle of fasting, we could possibly guide them to other Biblical principles they could put into practice in their homes, impacting future generations. We even had a song picked out for the event "Look What You've Done" by Tasha Layton. These events would have been life changing for attendees through praise, worship, story, and fellowship! But the opportunity to share our stories on that large of a scale hasn't happened yet.

Our mission statement at www.MeasureMeLife.com is to provide the tools necessary to launch and maintain a clean Intermittent Fasting lifestyle, enabling members to experience weight loss, increased confidence, spiritual growth, and overall wellness through our in-person and online support groups connecting "fasting friends" to one another for encouragement and fellowship.

Feeling like this was a pretty good mission, we joined our local Chamber of Commerce. We thought joining this local organization would give us a business foundation of support, but again we fell short as everyone would ask "so how are you going to make money with this business?" And I didn't know; we were just in the business of helping people! It didn't take long to be discouraged with the business side of MML. I wasn't clean fasting like I should, and the business was not at all what I had expected. But maybe that wasn't what the Lord had in HIS plans for us.

As I started writing my chapter for this book in February 2022, I didn't feel worthy of sharing my story. My story of weight loss, that is. I know, beyond a shadow of a doubt, that fasting works for me and can work for you. However, YOU must do IT, you must be consistently clean fasting daily! I have not been living my new lifestyle consistently the past six months and the weight is creeping back up towards the 220-pound mark. My husband, Brian, always tells our children during counsel, "The Good Lord gave us all free will - You are free to choose, but you aren't free from your choices and the consequences of those choices." I haven't gained all 45 pounds back, so that is a win for me, but the conviction is real; I haven't been practicing what I preach.

So, the best course of action was to announce to our Facebook® group that the Lives and in-person meetings would be canceled until further notice. My parents always say, "If you don't know what to do, do nothing at all." I've decided we will do nothing at all and BE STILL for a time. I do know this is my testimony and the way I am supposed to help people find a healthier lifestyle and Jesus, so I will not be defeated.

After that recent sermon and during writing my story, I have come to realize that I am the broken vase. I have been broken to pieces, ashamed, and discouraged, but I know a creator who is putting me back together emphasizing my flaws and imperfections to show the world my true, raw beauty.

Now, have I lost 80 pounds and kept it off for 36 months, nope, not yet! So, my story may not be what you would expect to read in a book about losing weight, but I have been very transparent in the struggles facing me daily. The story I am supposed to share is more about my spiritual awakening, healing, and self-acceptance. He wants me to know the number on the scale does NOT define me, and it does not define you; it is the relationship we have with our Heavenly Father that defines us and if you experience His grace and love, then you have GAINED everything!

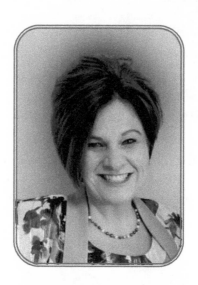

TAMMY ROACH

Tammy Roach and her amazingly supportive husband, Brian, has 4 adult children, Kate (Steve), Tyler (Katelynn), Samantha and Devin. She is a Bible Believing Christian and a member of Southeast Christian Church in Louisville, Kentucky, at the Bullitt County Campus. Tammy has worked as the Testing Services Director at the University of Louisville for over 30 years. Traveling with her husband is her favorite hobby, but she also enjoys crafting, event planning, and spending time with family and friends.

Shortly after starting Intermittent Fasting in October 2019 at 245 pounds, Tammy started a free online and in-person support group called Measure Me Life. The Facebook® group has grown to over 1,600 members and has recently transitioned to a small business, helping people worldwide connect to others in a Christian Intermittent Fasting community. Women, especially, have so many commitments we juggle that we NEED a community of others who can sympathize, empathize, and celebrate with us. Tammy is transparent and REAL in her everyday struggle to fast consistently, lose weight, and maintain the pounds she has lost. As you read her testimony, she declares she is a kintsugi vase in which God is highlighting her brokenness to create a more beautiful and unique woman than ever before.

For more information, go to www.MeasureMeLife.com or search for the group on YouTube® and Facebook®.

AFTERWORD

It is our sincere hope that these stories have not only caused you to think, but to ACT! As you read through the transformations, you have seen the authors experience many breakthroughs. We made a decision to change our lives. The common thread through all of our stories is that we chose not to stay stuck and made a decision to transform our lives through Intermittent Fasting.

May today be the day you are inspired to choose to create the life you deserve, be courageous enough to act, and surround yourself with inspirational and motivational people who want you to win.

Today is the perfect day to Take Action!

If any of these stories resonated with you, please connect with the authors. We are here to help you create the life you truly want to live.

With Gratitude,
Paige Davidson, Laurie Lewis, and Star McEuen

CPSIA information can be obtained
at www.ICGtesting.com
Printed in the USA
BVHW070959310522
638501BV00011B/573